A Fast Road to the Study of Emotions

Arne Vikan

A Fast Road to the Study of Emotions

An Introduction

Springer

Arne Vikan
Norwegian University of Science and Technology
Trondheim
Norway

ISBN 978-3-319-52312-5 ISBN 978-3-319-52313-2 (eBook)
DOI 10.1007/978-3-319-52313-2

Library of Congress Control Number: 2017945241

Printed on acid-free paper

This Springer imprint is published by Springer Nature
The registered company is Springer International Publishing AG
The registered company address is: Gewerbestrasse 11, 6330 Cham, Switzerland

This book is dedicated to my grandchildren:
Jørgen Vikan and Ulrik Vikan
Mikkel Westheim Vikan and Maiken Westheim Vikan

Preface

Scientists have prophesized that the present century will be the century for emotions. There are indications that this is already happening. The frequency of studies and theoretical views on emotions has shown a rapid increase since early in the 1990s and until today. Key terms for this is the relation between emotions and health, the significance of emotions for interaction and cooperation in the family, in the schools, and at work, and the mapping of emotions in the brain by the new magnetic resonance techniques. Scientists have even begun to show the satisfaction with life in different countries in terms of inhabitants' experiences of emotions such as happiness, sadness (depression) and anxiety. The media show, furthermore, a constant focus on emotions in news and interviews about politicians', actors', media- and sport persons' successes and failures, behaviors and intimate relationships, and in entertainment designed to arouse emotions, such as «idol» competitions and "reality TV".

The central reasons for the focus on emotions are that emotions are associated with human's basic competencies by being part of the foundations of thinking and communication. Emotional responses generate sufficient energy to register, experience, and become conscious of something, and are expressed and communicated in a flexible and visible facial area. They are indispensable and beneficial for our adaptation, but may function destructively and lead to personal and social conflicts and catastrophes.

Science should be guide for our emotional life as it is guide for our physical life and for a wide diversity of human coping and endeavors. This has not been established because research on emotions has been conducted within a number of different disciplines (e.g. anthropology, neuroscience, physiology, psychology, and sociology), and shows a traditional bias in focus on a few emotions (fear/anxiety, sadness/depression, and anger/aggression) dominated by theory and research either related to biological processes or to clinical (psychiatric) problems. A tendency toward an integrated view on emotions is, on the other hand, noticeable in the modern expansion of research into new areas of people's emotional experiences and emotional life.

The present book is written to support this integration tendency by presenting the main themes of scientific knowledge about emotions in 13 chapters. This is knowledge which should be is basic to those who prepare to (or are already engaged in) work that depends on the identification of people as being anxious, happy, angry, envious, shameful, disgusted, interested, etc., i.e. those whose duty is caring for people's health, are engaged in stimulating people to learn or achieve as individuals or in interaction, negotiate with people and help them select and make plans, and/or strive to control people's behavior to prevent them from harming themselves and others. The book is, consequently, directed at persons who are preparing for or is already working with persons and relationships, such as students and professionals in nursing, organizational- and economic professions, medicine, pedagogy, psychology, physiotherapy, and social work.

The book's Chap. 11 about historical background of research and recent theories, and Chap. 12 about the biological (neurological and physiological) basis of emotions represent frames which are traditionally the first chapters in an introductory text. These are often the first ones in an introductory book, and may well be read as the first ones in the present one for those who prefer to enter the subject from a distanced perspective. The priority for the present book was to get directly into the substantial knowledge, although prepared in Chap. 1 by a definition of emotions as a coordination of part, a description of their functioning as selective drivers, a discussion of research which indicate that emotions may serve as an unconscious early warning system and a short survey of emotion types and main emotions.

The first chapter is followed by Chap. 2 about the facial expressions and their universality, Chap. 3 about the experience, function, causes, and consequences of 13 emotions and Chap. 4 about the general experience of emotions and their intensity which may result in fears of emotion, the relation of emotions to the self, the tendency of emotional contagion and the need for sharing of emotion. Chapter 5 is a description of the development of emotions from birth, with a focus on the first year and the development of self-conscious emotions in the second- to fourth year, Chap. 6 is a presentation of how emotions both are influenced and influence cognition, and Chap. 7 comprises a discussion of indications that emotions are related to stress and health. The main factor in this respect may be the manner in which emotion is regulated, which is discussed in Chap. 8 about emotion regulation, which also is involved and may be part of emotional work and intelligence discussed in Chap. 10. All themes related to emotional life may show variation pertaining to the set of values, beliefs, and social organization which is implied in the concept of culture as is shown in Chap. 9. The final Chap. 13 in the book is reserved for an overview and notes on a few themes which had to be ignored in the ordinary chapters.

The term «emotion» is used consistently as the central term rather than «feelings» in this book. One reason for this is that "emotion" has its root from «emovere» in Latin. "Emovere" refers to being moved by something, and is an intrinsic and typical quality of the phenomena we ordinarily refer to as emotions. Other reasons for using "emotion" throughout the book are that "emotion" is a central term in many worldwide languages (English, French, Spanish, and Portuguese), and is the main word which employed in research on the subject. In most headings "emotions" is preferred to the more conservative "emotion". This is because the subject of this book is a family of functional forms with common basic characteristics who differ in experience, facial expression and behaviors.

Emotions refer to people's behavior and manner of living their life. The best way to learn from the presented book is, therefore, to relate the results from the cited research to one's own life. An attempt to facilitate this is made in the present book by a challenge to reflect on themes or issues by two reflection questions at the end of each chapter. Each chapter also ends with proposals for 2–3 research projects. The majority of these are rather straightforward, but they have scientific merit only to the extent to which they fulfill the requirements of reliability, validity, and representation.

The book started as a project on children's socio-emotional development with support from the Norwegian Non-Fiction Writers' and Translators' Association, and was enlarged and based on a course on emotions for doctoral students at the Universidade Federal da Paraiba, Joao Pessoa, Brazil in 2013/2014 when the author was a visiting professor as Bolsista CAPES. The author is indebted to CAPES for the opportunity to develop a book based on the course and published in Norwegian on "Akademika Forlag" (ISBN 978-82-321-0263-1) in 2014 with the title "Innføring om emosjoner". The present book is a translation of the Norwegian text with an additional chapter (Chap. 10) on emotions at the workplace and with several improvements after suggestion from Springer's reviewers. Thanks are due to my wife Anne-Lise Løvaas and to Tom Knudsen at the Institute of Psychology NTNU for great help in preparing the manuscript.

Trondheim, Norway
Summer 2017

Arne Vikan

Contents

What Are Emotions?

1

Teil I

This chapter is focused on the definition, measurement, function, and causes of emotions. The chapter begins with the central concept that an emotion is not a substance but a coordination of processes, and is defined as a coordination of experiences, behavioral expressions and physiological/neurological components. The function of emotions is described as selective and motivating, and emotions, therefore, can be conceived as selective drivers. Causes of emotions are shown as cognitive and conscious, but results from studies show that they may also be unconsciously triggered from subcortical parts of the brain and function as early warning signals. This suggests that emotions may be differently dependent on biological and social factors corresponding to "basic" and "social" emotional types. A list of ten basic emotions is cited at the end of the chapter.

1.1 Main Concept

The word «emotion» is one of several words which refer to similar responses, such as «feeling», "affect" and "mood". There are no clear-cut differences between the references of these words, and they are, therefore, of little use to this book. The word "emotion" will consequently be used as a unitary concept, but "feeling" and "to feel" will be used when this is indicated by the context.

1.2 Substantial Unit or Coordination of Components?

Emotions are different from reactions which are directly based on sensations such as pain and temperature variations (warmth and cold), and needs such as hunger and thirst. Emotions vary in qualitative types (happy, sad, afraid, etc.) and in intensity from mild to very intense such as from ordinary fear and anger to, respectively, nightmares and rage. But what is their content, what do they consist of?

Imagine the last time you were clearly angry or afraid. You may remember that you perceived and thought something, and that there was something that you did or was very tempted to do. You probably also noticed changes in your body, for instance that your breath was more forced and/or that muscles in your stomach, arms and legs became tense. This tells you that an emotion is not a simple "feeling" but something that consists of different parts or components. Three main components of emotions are distinguished: Experience, physiological reactions, and behavior. The 6–7 most common emotions also entail a typical facial expression.

Figure 1.1 (see page 2) shows three emotions which can be used as examples. Notice that each emotion concerns something important for Mary, John and Silvia. This is a basic characteristic. Emotions indicate the experience that we are aroused by something which is important and has significance for our life.

The first of the three components of emotion refers to Mary, John, and Silvia's experience of, respectively, fear, happiness, and interest. It may be that perception and responses are so fast that Mary is aware of her fear only after the truck has passed by. And that Silvia needs to consider for a moment before she agrees that her interest for music is an emotion. But the experience of an emotion is clearly present in both instances. There may be different experiences of each emotion, such as for instance between Mary's fear of being hit by the truck and her fear when she perceives a snake at a distance, but both experiences includes a quality of fear. It is this quality which provides the emotional «color» of an experience.

The two other components of the emotion are related to Mary, John, and Silvia's behavior. One component is the specific behaviors and facial expressions of each emotion. The other is the arousal of the body which is implied by the behavior. The arousal refers to physiological- and neurological reactions which are released when an emotion is activated. The breath in Mary's fear is for instance increased to get more oxygen, the heart is stimulated to beat faster to drive blood faster to the muscles, and the muscles are tensed for immediate action (see Sects. 7.2 and 12.2.2 for detailed descriptions). Arousal reactions of an emotion can be similar in a wide variety of behaviors. Anger may, for instance, be aroused to the same extent when one is complaining about a TV program at home, argues against someone at work or fails in some outdoor game. The physiological reactions may be the reason that emotional experiences often are referred to as "emotional tension".

A. Vikan, *A Fast Road to the Study of Emotions*,
DOI 10.1007/978-3-319-52313-2_1

Teil I

Fig. 1.1 Three examples of emotions

Mary: Fear

Mary is about to cross a street while she is preoccupied in thoughts about a friend. She does not notice a truck which is approaching fully loaded and in high velocity until it is very near with screeching brakes. Then she is filled with a sudden and intense fear and reacts immediately by jumping backwards and manages to avoid being hit by just an inch

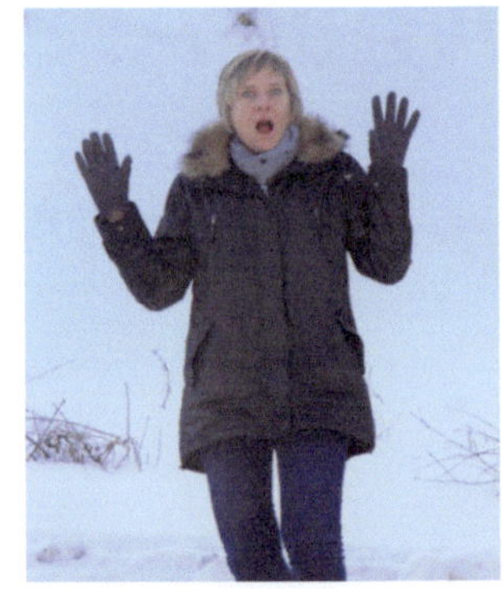

John: Happiness

John is informed on his cell that he has received the top mark at an important examination. He experiences warmth in his body and smiles all over his face. After some time he becomes restless, walks about then he calls his parents and his friends with a voice so shaky of happiness that they have difficulty in understanding what he says. His happiness continues through the rest of the day and during the night when he goes to a party and dances his happiness until the sun raises the next morning.

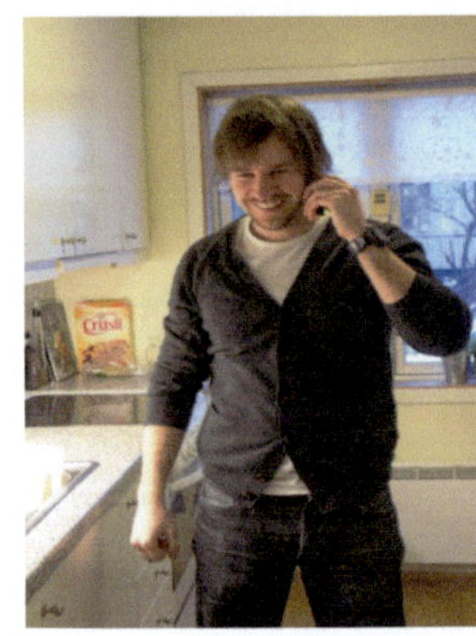

Silvia: Interest

Silvia has been interested in country music as long as she can remember. At first she was only focusing on the tunes, but after some time she began to notice all the different bands and vocalists. After that she began to use her PC to get information about the history of the music from different regions and countries, and when she began her studies at the University country music became the subject for her Master's thesis.

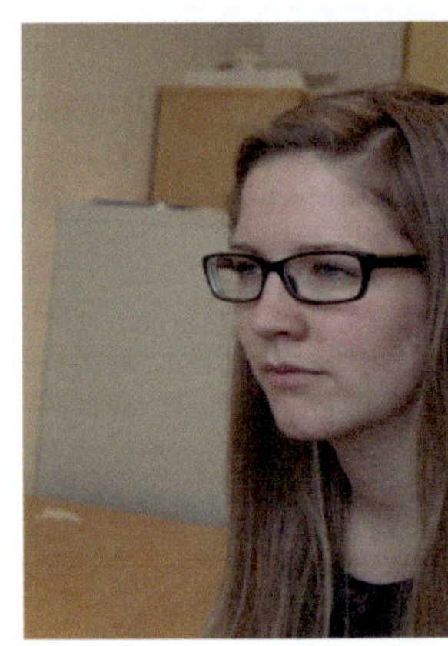

Many scientists held that emotions are always linked to behavior. They point out that behavior is present in terms of an action readiness even though a specific behavior is not present. This will also be shown in a physiological arousal. "Behavior" in this instance is enacted as work on the inside of the body. Thus, a person may be on her/his sofa with intense non-manifest emotions (sadness or anger) all day long and be exhausted in the afternoon. He or she may even be unaware of this internal work and cannot understand that he or she are extremely tired after "having done nothing the whole day".

Mary, John and Silvia's facial expressions in Fig. 1.1 are all typical of an emotion, and may be considered as facial «signatures» which are evident across the variation in their emotional behavior. John's expression of happiness in Fig. 1.1 will for instance show much variation during the day and the afternoon, but the signature of happiness will be evident in frequent and similar smiles. The signature of Mary's fear is wide open eyes and an open mouth, and Silvia's signature of interest is focused eyes and somewhat knitted eyebrows. The expression may show variation between the millions of persons who experience these emotions, but the facial signature will be recognized in all instances. This is discussed further in the next chapter.

The three main components are shown in Fig. 1.2 (see page 3). It is important to keep in mind that an emotion is a coordination or

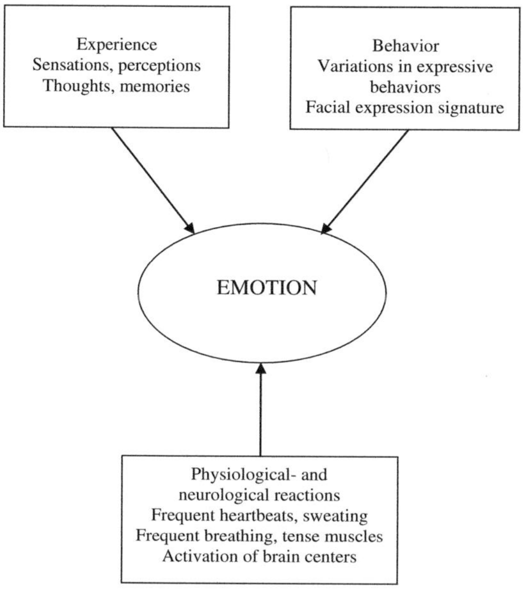

Fig. 1.2 The three main components of emotion

composite of components. The specific situational experiences and behaviors of an emotion may vary greatly, but the coordination of components that comprise the emotion will be the same. The coordination will also stay stable although the saliency of each component may vary between persons. Some persons may for instance experience strong physiological sensations, such as tensions in the stomach, head or the breast area, while others may scarcely notice any such internal signals. And some emotions, such as disgust and fear, are associated with much more marked sensations than interest and guilt, which seem to be only very lightly related to physiological responses (see Sect. 4.1.1).

1.3 Definition of Emotion

Definitions are necessary to establish confidence that we are talking about the same thing or concept. An unequivocal definition has been difficult to obtain because researchers have focused definitions on one- or two of the three emotional components. This has led to many discussions were researchers have been talking past- rather than to each other. A realization that the definition must comprise all three components has emerged in the recent 15–20 years. What seems to remain is to incorporate the variable of time into the definition. Examples of this variation are shown in Fig. 1.1, where Mary's fear only last for a few seconds, whereas John's and Silvia's emotions lasts for days, months and even for years. Several studies have shown that 2/3 of participants have rated the duration of their emotional episodes as more than one hour. 31% of participants in one of these studies held that their emotions could last for more than a day (Frijda, 2007). A definition of emotions according to this and to the three-component description is as follows: "*An emotion is a coordination or composite of experiences, behavioral expressions and physiological/neurological components with varying duration.*"

1.4 Measuring Emotions

There is no measurement directly related to the three-component definition of emotions. Measurement has, consequently, been based on one of the three main components, and serves as indication rather than as direct expression of emotions. Descriptions of specific methods will be supplied in this book mainly in relation to presentation of studies and research areas.

Measurement of emotions raises several problems for research. Emotions are difficult to find when they are needed for scrutiny, they are not very stable in time, and they are difficult to record or observe in ways that do not influence the measurement itself. Researchers have developed a variety of procedures and techniques to cope with these problems (see Coan & Allen, 2007). Persons can for instance be stimulated to be emotional by using hypnosis, suggestive music and/or arousing films/videos. Electronic methods are developed to identify and register emotions based on facial expressions. Very light instruments have been developed to measure physiological reactions without distracting the person which is being measured. And modern magnetic resonance imagining (fMRI) and positron emission tomography (PET), which make direct registration of cerebral activity, have opened vast possibilities for research on how the brain affects and is affected by emotions.

1.5 Functions of Emotions: Selective Drivers

Why do emotions exist? What may be their tasks? The answer is that emotions are part of the adaptation to the environment. Mary in Fig. 1.1 avoids being run over and quite possible killed because her perception of a threat is linked to an arousal of muscle activation and behavior which results in an immediate avoidance of the deathly peril. The fear emotion saves her. Notice that this shows a coordination of the components in Fig. 1.2 which mobilizes energy that serves as a drive to select the appropriate behaviors.

It has been a dominating conception since Darwin's (1872) pioneering work that emotions are developed over millions of years to serve the survival of the species. This does not refer specifically to the human species. Withdrawal from danger, attraction and approach to safety and nurturing circumstances, and aggressive behavior in order to obtain some necessary good is shown by all animals and possibly by many creatures outside the animal kingdom as well. Darwin held, for example, that emotions are readily shown in insects. The main point here is that emotions are identified as universal functional forms which characterize organisms' adaptation to their environments.

The selective and driving aspects of emotions can be elaborated further by reference to Tomkins' (1962, 1963) interpretations that emotions are motivational systems. Motivation is a dynamical factor in the adaptation. It «drives» humans to make plans and to behave in order to obtain something which is associated with positive emotions, such as being happy or proud, and to avoid negative emotions, such as being afraid, sad or shameful. Motivation is also part of emotions in terms of their expressive behaviors. Examples of this are shown in the behaviors of all protagonists in Fig. 1.1. These behaviors are also examples of selectivity. John shows for instance his emotional selectivity by engaging in happy mannerisms (rather than eating or reading something), and by contacting his friends and propose a celebration during the night (rather than going to bed), while Silvia shows selectivity by (i.e.) access various sites on the internet and to stay at the library to research books on music in different countries (rather than to play volley-ball or to hang out with friends).

Emotional selectivity is also evident in the registration and active attention to stimuli. A person which is afraid is extremely tense and is constantly on the look-out for indications of danger in the surroundings. A happy person is only focusing on positive stimuli which can contribute to sustain her/his happiness. An angry person is locked at a target for aggression. One may represent this selective function as a camera which takes emotionally colored pictures. The fear, happiness, and anger pictures will then be three very different pictures of the same environment.

Examples and results of the selective drive are that emotions are established in the evolution as specific reactions or patterns of reactions to specific stimuli (carnivorous animals, attractive partners, and venomous food), combination of stimuli (resistance, loss) and the relation between the organism and the environment. Selective reactions can ensure a stable adaptation because the organism's energy is directed to the central aspects of the environment. They save the organism from reacting to new stimuli that are constantly encountered, and serve as a basis for prediction and control. The functional value of this selective drive system is shown in persons who have managed to suppress their emotions. They seem to have lost the energy and color in their lives. They feel that they lack content and direction, they are scarcely able to want something for themselves, they have large problems in choosing among alternatives, and they experience their existence as grey and with lack of meaning.

1.6 Causes of Emotions and the Question of Consciousness

External stimulation or events, such as the car, the top mark, and the music in Fig. 1.1, are the most clear and probably most frequent causes of emotions. Causes are also frequently internal and subjective in terms of thoughts and memories. In these cases they may be difficult to notice and to know, and persons may experience emotions without being aware of their causes. Two examples of internal causes are shown in Table 1.1.

Links between emotions and their causes are systematic and forms part of emotional selectivity. There are variations between persons, but most persons, even from different cultures, are afraid, happy, angry, sad, shameful or proud for the same reasons and/or events and influences (see Chap. 9). This refers to our awareness and attention to a stimulus because of its significance or meaning. Meaning, for instance that something may be threatening, attractive, or challenging, becomes a releaser of emotions. This also pertains to the internal causes in Fig. 1.1. Mark and Sally became aware of, respectively, a bird and a car that led to respective thoughts of a girlfriend and a father with associated meanings which released the emotions of, respectively sadness and anxiety. A causal sequence for emotions indicated by this is shown in Fig. 1.3 (see page 5).

The model implies that we must be aware of something before we can be with an emotion. Awareness is included in attention, experiences, perception, associations and thoughts, which all are referred to as «cognitive processes» or just «cognition». The causation model is, accordingly, a cognitive model. This model is domineering, and might be conceived as a norm of emotional causation, but it is not the only possible one. An objection to the cognitive model is that emotions often seem just to be present, or, in Zajonc's (1980) words: "Preferences need no inferences". We do not necessarily experience a specific cause of an emotion. We may be sad or anxious without being aware of a cause like Mark and Sally, but unlike them we may not be able to identify any cause even with help.

Another objection to the cognitive model is that emotions at times only are based on a direct response to a stimulus without any meaning being involved. Mary's immediate response to the threat in Table 1.1 is an example of this. The objections are met by argumentation from the cognitive appraisal viewpoint

Table 1.1 Two examples of causes of emotions

Mark
Mark was aware of a mild sadness the whole day without knowing why. In the afternoon he reflected on this, and remembered that he had seen a small yellow bird outside his window when he had breakfast. It reminded him that he had seen exactly the same when he had breakfast with a former girlfriend two years ago. He had loved her, but she had broken up the relationship that same year. Mark became sad when he remembered this, but he was late for work, had to hurry and was distracted from his memories. But the sadness remained
Sally
Sally suffered from frequent anxiety attacks which did not seem to have a cause. When her therapist asked for an example she said she had felt a sudden intense anxiety the other day when leaving the shopping center to pick up her car. She was alone, everything was calm and there was no cause of anxiety. When asked to explore her thoughts when she went to the parking she remembered that she had seen a car which was similar to her father's. This had led to thoughts that he was nearby and that she risked meeting him. The thoughts were very discomforting and were immediately suppressed and left her with an anxiety without reasonable cause

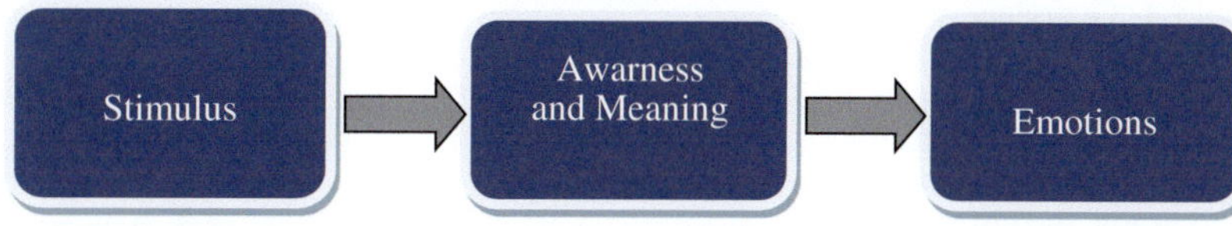

Fig. 1.3 Causal sequence of emotions

(see Chap. 6) that cognition may be unconsciously performed as an extremely fast and very simple process of registering whether a stimulus is positive or negative. This leads further to a question if emotions are always conscious, which may seem as a contradiction in terms since experience, i.e. awareness, is one of emotions' the main components.

1.7 Unconscious Emotions. Øhman and Soares' (1994) Study

Many will agree that emotions can be unconscious. They can supply examples of persons who show all signs of envy, jealousy, or being in love, and who deny this vehemently when this is pointed out to them. This is, however, examples of suppression and/or reluctance to accept that one feels these emotions. The examples do not show anything about the causes of these emotions, or how they are aroused.

A well-known study related to a question about unconscious emotions was conducted by Øhman and Soares (1994) with 16 students in each of three groups as participants: Persons with snake phobia, persons with spider phobia and non-phobic persons. The study was administered in a laboratory in front of a PC. Participants were informed that they would be shown pictures of a flower, a mushroom, a snake, and a spider. One picture of each object was then shown in 30 ms, which is too short for the picture to be remembered afterwards. The pictures were presented both in an open and a masked procedure. The open procedure consisted simply of a 30 ms presentation followed by a recognition test of pictures. The masked procedure consisted of showing the picture of a non-experimental picture for 100 ms immediately after the 30 ms presentation of the experimental picture. This procedure is called "bachward masking". Backward masking is employed to block afterimages of a picture, i.e. images of a stimulus which may continue a short time after the stimulus is removed.

Participants' emotional reactions were indicated by variation in the skin's electric conductance in terms of the Galvanic Skin Response (GSR) measure, and by a rating of awareness of the stimulus. The GSR registers electric skin conductance stimulated by sweating, and is an indicator of emotional reaction because sweating which is triggered by emotional arousal. A common measurement is made by a tiny electrode in a Velcro strap at the tip of the index and the middle finger. Several examples of this can be encountered by search for "GSR measurement with finger electrodes" on the Internet (see Sect. 12.2).

Awareness of emotion was measured by participants' identification after the presentation of each picture which picture they thought they had seen, and by ratings of the extent to which they experienced arousal, negative tension and lack of control. Rating was made after each picture by marking on nine-point scales from «not at all» to «very much» for each of the three experiential dimensions arousal, tension, and control. An overview of the study is shown in Table 1.2.

Øhman and Soares did a pilot run before the critical experiments which showed that there was no difference in participants' ability (or lack of ability) to identify objects on pictures after 30 ms exposure. The experimental results indicated in Table 1.2 was that the non-phobic participants showed indication of arousal neither for masked nor for open presentations of objects. No picture was evidently registered as sufficiently important (see Sect. 1.2) to trigger an emotional response. The results from the phobic groups were strikingly different: GSR measures were markedly and differentially elevated show, i.e. the snake-phobic participants showed very high GSRs to the picture of a snake, and the spider-phobic participants showed very high GSRs to the picture of the spider. These specific responses were shown in both the open and the masked condition together with a general elevation of GSRs for the other pictures in comparison to the non-phobic group in the masked condition. The GSR from the phobic participants thus may show some heightened "suspicion" or "sensitivity", but the main point is that their differentiated response to masked stimuli showed that they were aroused by stimulation they could not experience or being aware of. The test for awareness corroborated the assumption that the content of the pictures could not be recognized, whereas the ratings showed parallel variations to those from the GSR measures.

Many subsequent studies have shown similar results to those of Øhman and Soares (1994). It has, however, been argued that the demonstration of unconscious registration of the stimulus

Table 1.2 Overview of Øhman and Soares' (1994) study

Set-up: Participants were shown pictures of a flower, a mushroom, a snake, and a spider on a PC screen
Participants: 16 each in a group of students with snake phobia, spider phobia, and persons without an anxiety diagnosis
Procedure: Each picture was shown in 30 ms, one time in an open condition (not followed by another picture) and one time in a masked condition (immediately followed by exposure in 100 ms of a neutral picture)
Measure: GSR and rating of experience of each picture
Results: None of the students could recognize the exposed picture afterwards Variation in GSR and ratings only shown in phobic students, and was largest for the picture which corresponded to the phobia

Teil I

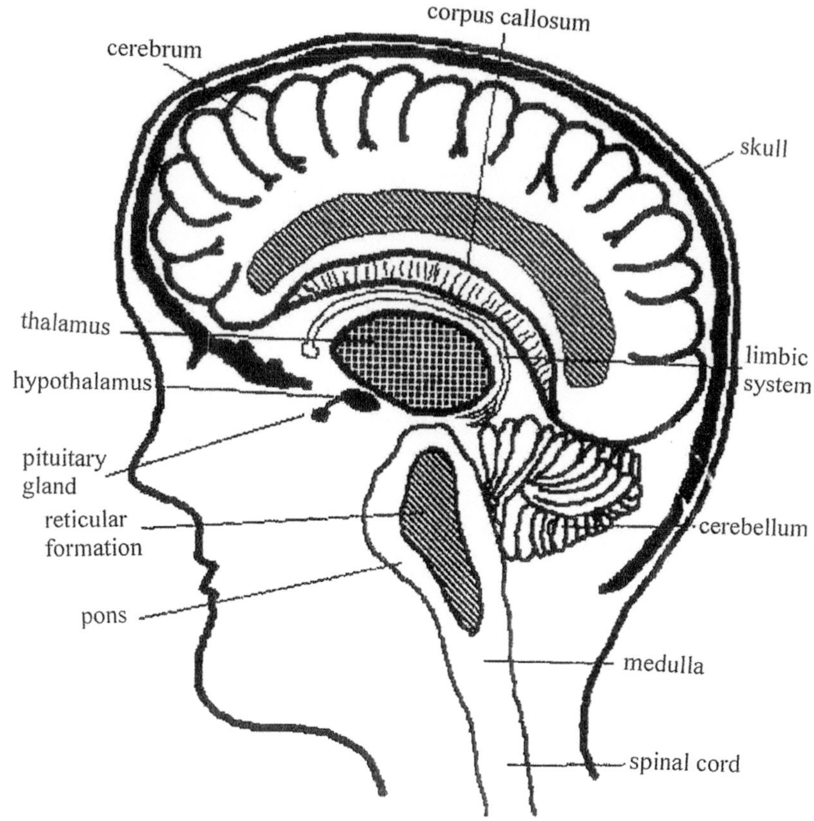

Fig. 1.4 Overview which shows the cortex on top of the corpus callosum and the sub-cortical structures thalamus, hypothalamus and limbic system

pictures in this study showed that participants were unaware of the causes of emotions but not that they were unaware of the actual emotions. A more direct test in relation to this argument was a study where participants' were served drinks and ask to judge their value after having attended to masked happy and angry faces. Emotional responses were shown in this study as differences in behavior and evaluation depending on the stimulus they had attended to, i.e. by more drinking and positive judgments after happy than angry stimuli. These participants did not report a specific emotional experience, and they therefore seemed to be influenced by an emotion that they were not aware of (Winkielman, Berridge, & Wilbarger, 2005).

Researchers agree that the causes and experience of emotions may be out of reach for consciousness. The unconscious causation may be sensations from smell, taste, hearing and/or vision that informs on the environment. The processing of information can take place outside of consciousness because it is performed subcortically, i.e. based on other parts of the brain than the cortex, who supports language, thought and conscious reflection. The subcortical part comprises basic sections of the brain which is shared by animals and humans and which was developed hundreds of millions of years before the evolution of humankind. A simplified sketch of the brain in Fig. 1.4 shows the cerebrum, which contains the cortex, the corpus callosum, which connects the two hemispheres, and the subcortical limbic system with thalamus and hypothalamus on top of the spinal cord with the medulla and the reticular formation.

1.8 A Subcortical Early Warning System

The indications of unconscious causation point to a subcortical anchoring of emotions. This is confirmed by observations that emotions are present in children who are born without neocortex (encephalic) and in adults with damaged cortex. Confirmation is also shown in results from registration of variations in the blood-flow of the brain by fMRI and in animal experimentation. This establishes a neurological background for the concept of emotion as evolutionary selective drivers of adaptation. A further interpretation may be that emotions have their evolutionary root as an early, subcortical warning system in the brain. It is this system who saves Mary's life in Table 1.1, and which Ekman (1994) referred to when he proposed that emotions are aroused so fast that they are present before we are aware that they have been triggered. And it is because of this system that we often conceive of emotions as something that happens to us which we have not chosen and which we may not be fully responsible for.

The subcortical reactions can, furthermore, confirm a concept of emotions as neurological circuits or programs in the DNA. This was a main part of Darwin's (1872) theory which we referred to in Sect. 1.5, and which will be elaborated further in Chaps. 2 and 11. Other evidence for the theory is that the facial expression for a group of emotions seem to be the same

Fig. 1.5 Non-cognitive causal sequence of emotional experience

in people around the world (see Chap. 2), that emotions are shown and recognized by infants (see Chap. 5), and by results which indicate that different emotions are related to specific parts of the brain (see Chap. 12). Modern concepts in the same direction are interpretations that emotions are related to a constant activity in the brain of balancing the organism's processes and states internally and in relation to stimulation from the environment (Damasio, 1994, 1999; Panksepp & Biven, 2012; see also Izard's and Russell and Feldman Barrett's theories in Chap. 11). Emotions in these theories are patterns of activity which is released because of an imbalance where the organism is weighted toward something which is seen as important to its survival (e.g. the sight of a dangerous animal) which means that some response (e.g. withdrawal) must be initiated. Notice that cognition (awareness) results from the first emotional reactions when the experience follows a subcortical registration. These reactions can be considered as emotional components which lead to an emotional experience, and which in turn forms a different sequence of reactions than those included in the cognitive model and which are suggested in Fig. 1.5.

Other examples of non-cognitive reactions as triggers of emotions are that emotions can be aroused by electric stimulation in brain areas and by centrally stimulating chemicals in terms of cocaine and heroin. This type of stimulation is a main source of emotions in research within affective neuroscience. We will not cite from this important area except for a general sketch of neuropsychological research on emotions in Chap. 12. The reason for this is that affective neuroscience has been dominated by research on animals and by components of only a few emotions (mainly fear and anger).

1.9 Basic and Social Emotions

Indications of subcortical reactions and universal expressions in support of Darwin's theory have led many researchers to propose that emotions are inherited. Others have protested, pointed to the cognitive model of causation of emotions and argued that emotions comprise experiences and behavior which only can be learnt during childhood. This argument is often extended to comprise the fact that emotions such as shame, guilt and envy have not been associated with either subcortical reactions or with universal expressions.

Controversies whether emotions are inherited or learned forms, and whether they are influenced mainly by biological- or social factors will pop up in several parts of this book.

One aspect of the discussions is that it seems to have reached a consensus that some emotions are mainly dominated by biological- and others by social factors. This can serve as a differentiation of biologically basic- and social emotions, where basic emotions are defined by specific facial expressions, motivation (goals), experience, and behavior, and shows signs of being managed by neurological programs ("hardwiring") (Ackerman, Abe & Izard, 1998; Izard & Ackerman, 2000).

The highest agreement on the definition as basic emotions has been reached for happiness, interest, fear, surprise, anger, disgust and sadness. But "basic" does not mean that emotional components are not influenced by the environment. Changes in the experience and expression of all these emotions are shown during childhood and adolescence. Children seem to attain emotional responses which are similar to the adult forms when they are about one year of age, which shows that it can be differentiated between infants' native basic emotions and the ordinary form of the emotions which seem to be developed at the end of the child's first year (see Chap. 5).

The group of social emotions includes generally shame, guilt and pride, which are also often classified as «self-conscious emotions». Envy and jealousy are other candidates for a social emotions classification. None of the social emotions can be associated with universally agreed facial expressions, but attempts at describe characteristic patterns of facial expressions, bodily postures, and behavior have sometimes been proposed for some of these emotions. All of them seem to be present in human cultures, and they imply physiological reactions which can be detected by GSR and other physiological measures. The social emotions seem to be present from the last part of the child's second year (shame) to the third (guilt and shame) and fourth (envy and jealousy) year of life (see Chap. 5), and shows large cultural variations in expression and causality.

There will probably always be controversies as regards the classification of emotions. An example may be Carroll Izard, who has been doing emotion research for more than 40 years and has proposed several different lists of basic emotions. An example is the sample of emotions which were discussed in Izard (1991) and is depicted in Table 1.3.

Izard (2007, 2009) has proposed a revised list where "surprise" is excluded because it seems to be part of "interest", and "shame", "guilt" and "contempt" excluded because of a lack

Table 1.3 Sample of emotions

Interest
Happiness
Surprise
Sadness
Anger
Disgust
Contempt
Fear
Shame
Guilt

From Izard (1991)

of indications of associations to a neurological program and of universal facial expressions (see Sect. 11.4.1). The emotions in Table 1.3 can be conceived as a reasonable sample of important emotions, and will be referred to later in the book.

1.10 Practical Relevance

This chapter has been an introduction which may suggest several applications of emotional concepts and measurement. This will be elaborated further in the following chapters in this book. A direct suggestion based on the concept of emotions as aroused by something which is important and has significance for us. The implication is our emotions points to the directions we must follow to comply with Socrates' call to know oneself in order to be a full human being.

A beginning can be made by using Izard's list in Table 1.3 to do systematic rating of one's emotional responses. One may for instance rate how often (e.g. from «less than one time each week» to «several times each day»), lasting (e.g. from "less than five minutes" to "more than an hour") and intensely (e.g. from "very mildly" to "very intensely") one has experienced each emotion the last month (or week). This emotional mapping can be supplied by noting the causes which could be associated to the arousal of the different emotions.

A further elaboration of self-knowledge can be made by rating the frequency, duration, and intensity in relation to one's significant other persons. This may provide several new perspectives on one's relationships, and indicate how each of them be developed further.

1.11 Summary

An emotion is defined in this book as a "*coordination or composite of experiences, behavioral expressions and physiological/neurological components with varying duration.*"

The processes involved comprise work (expenditure of energy) in terms of physiological arousal which is focused on the body's adjustment efforts by leading to selective experiences and driving selectively (motivating) for the specific behaviors.

The causes of emotions are most often cognitive, which means that it is related to the perception, awareness and attribution of meaning to something. Results from Øhman and Soares's (1994) study have, however, suggested that emotions also can be unconsciously aroused from processes in the subcortical part of the brain. The subcortical processing means that emotions can be an evolutionary early warning system of threats and challenges to the organism's adaptation, and may be caused by biological rather than cognitive factors.

A group of 6–7 emotions conform to characteristics of basic emotions by including specific experience, motivation, and behavior, showing universal facial expression and being present in infants. These emotions seem to be mainly biologically anchored. A second sample of 4–5 emotions show great variation in expression, is present later (from the last half of the child's second year) in development, and are called «social emotions» because their primary anchoring seem to be in social relationships.

Reflection Questions

1. Examples of selective drive: Imagine yourself in a public park when you suddenly see something that make you interested, happy, angry or afraid. What are the instigated thoughts, behaviors and physiological reactions for each of the emotions?
2. Indications of unconscious emotions: Responses you have done without understanding why, sudden realization that your behavior in some context or to some person is motivated by a specific emotion, and reluctance to do something without understanding why.

Research/Exercise Examples

1. Which notes in the present day's news (paper and net) refer directly or indirectly to emotions?
2. Establish a measure of "emotional investment" or "emotional appeal" (discuss these concepts) by using a three-point rating of "not at all—to some extent—definitively" with points assigned, respectively, as 0–1–2. Have all persons in your study group rate the existence of each of the emotions in Table 1.3 in relation to well-known persons (or to all members of the group). The sum of points for all ratings divided by number of raters will show mean investment/appeal for each emotion, and may also be merged to a measure of "emotionality" generally, and/or to measures of "positive" and "negative" emotionality" (see Chap. 3).

Further Reading

Ekman, P., & Davidson, R. J. (Eds.). (1994). *The nature of emotion. Fundamental questions*. Oxford, UK: Oxford University Press.

Feldman Barret, L. F., Niedenthal, P. M., & Winkielman, P. (Eds.). (2005). *Emotion and consciousness*. New York: The Guilford Press.

Frijda, N. H. (2007). *The laws of emotion*. Mahwah, NJ: Erlbaum.

Facial Expressions

2

Teil I

The human face has a main role in theory and research on emotions. A background for this is provided in Chap. 2 by a presentation of the characteristics of the face and a description of Charles Darwin's pioneering views on the function of the facial expressions and their significance for emotions. The chapter comprises sketches of the facial expressions of basic emotions and indications that these expressions may lead by facial feedback to emotional experiences. This leads further to a question of the universality of facial expressions and to a description of Ekman's central studies. The last part of Chap. 2 comprise a discussion of results from a study where persons seemed to be unconsciously imitating other's facial expressions of emotions in ways that suggest a neural mirroring of emotional activation and that emotions may be contagious.

2.1 The Human Face

When you look for emotions in your surroundings they are primarily visible in persons' faces. Actually, this is a practice you have engaged in since you were born. Studies have shown that newborns prefer to look at human faces to other types of stimulation. This may be because the face is a closed form which is easy to grasp, and which is rich in information from contours, symmetrical details and movement. When exploring the face with their eyes newborns inspect mainly the contour of the hair. The inspection of the details of the face starts about a month and a half after birth, with eyes and eyebrows as the preferred targets. Faces, and primarily that of the mother and the father, are the dominating, and possibly the only important, visual stimulus during the first six months of the infant's life (Stern, 1977).

There are several other reasons than visual qualities which attract attention to the face. The face is used when we satisfy our basic needs. We breathe with our nose and we eat and drink through our mouth, and we bolster our security by picking up information from long distances with our eyes and ears. And the face is the source for our use of sounds and language to communicate and interact with other persons. Thus, it is the face we use when we signalize threats, friendliness, disgust, anger and interest, and when we gather information from others.

The importance of the face can be underlined by the fact that evolution has established a specific area for face recognition in the brain. The area is called "fusiform gyrus" and is located in the temporal lobe in the neocortex (see Chap. 11). Persons who have been injured in this area can get «prosopagnosia», which means that they are no longer able to recognize other person's faces.

2.2 The Facial Expressions

Specific facial expressions of emotions such as happiness, anger, and fear are formed by a thin elastic layer of skin fitted on top of an outer and an inner layer of 20 striate muscles. The outer layer consists of many small muscles which influence changes in the forehead (brow), around the eyes and eyebrows and in the mouth and corners of the mouth. The inner layer comprises larger muscles that influence movement in the jaws. Some less used muscles stimulate movements around the nostrils and the ears. Several detailed descriptions of facial muscles can be available by a search for "Facial muscles" and Facial muscles of emotion" on the Internet.

Several attempts at mapping the relations between muscles and facial expressions were made before Charles Darwin presented the results from his studies in 1872. Eight chapters in this book comprise descriptions of 37 emotions and emotional states as well as references to the active muscles which were involved in each case. This was followed up by Tomkins' theory and by studies by Ekman, Izard and the Swedish professor of anatomy Carl-Herman Hjortsjø in the 1960s.

The aim of the mapping was to arrive at exact depictions of the activation of the muscles related to changes in parts of the face for each emotion. Such descriptions can be an objective measure of emotional arousal and a method to identify the type of emotion in each case. There is a pragmatic significance of this which can be associated with the emotional characteristic of selective drivers (see Sect. 1.5). Anger «drives» for instance a person toward direct or indirect aggression, fear to attempts to hide and/or to distract attention to oneself, and sadness to resignation and passivity. This means that nurses, medical doctors, psychologists, psychotherapists, teachers etc. may

A. Vikan, *A Fast Road to the Study of Emotions*,
DOI 10.1007/978-3-319-52313-2_2

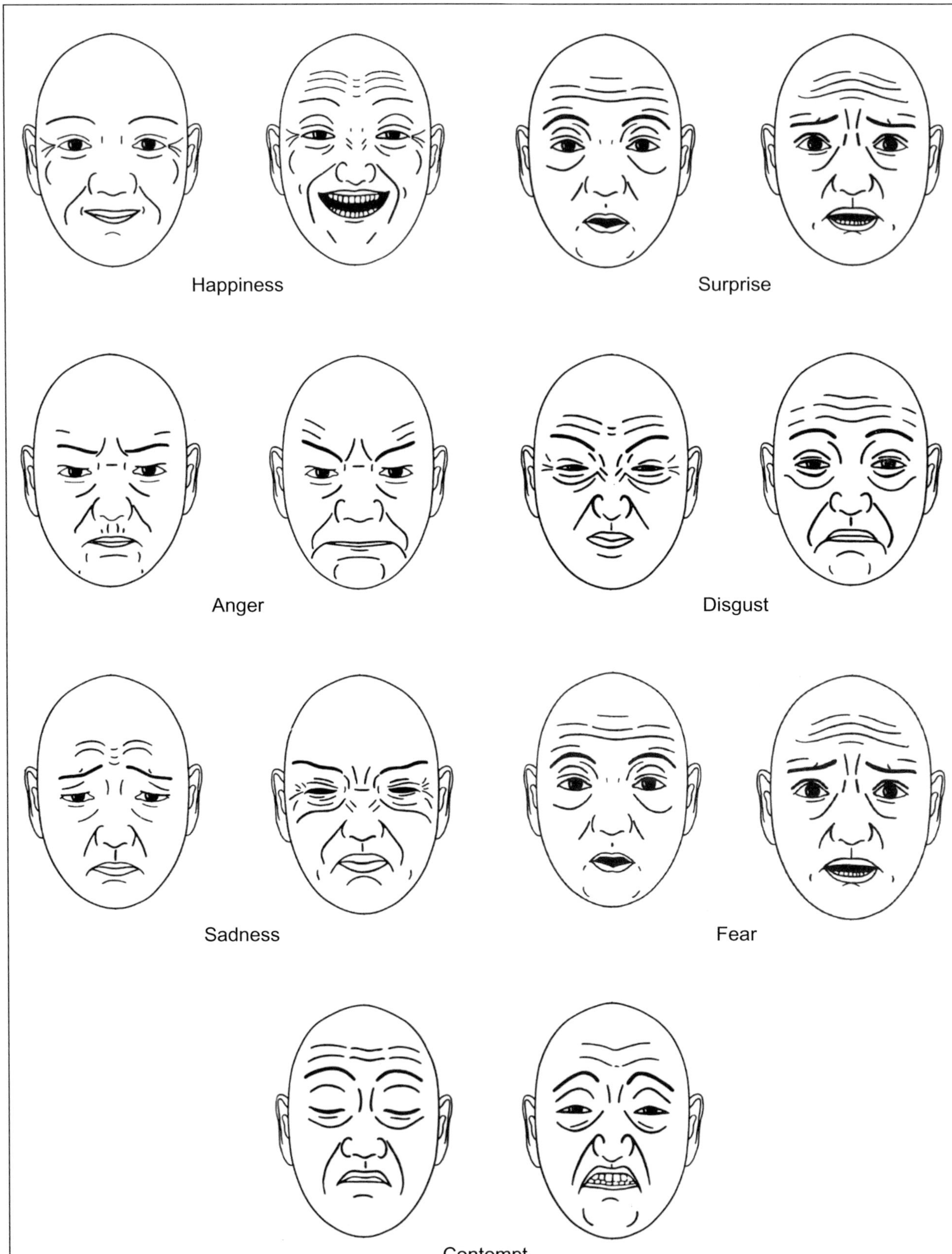

Fig. 2.1 Schematic facial expressions of mild (*left*) and intense (*right*) examples of seven emotions (from Hjortsjø, 1969)

Table 2.1 Description of facial expressions of nine emotions

Emotion	Description
Interest	Eyebrows lifted and slightly drawn together, eyes follow an object, mouth slightly open and lips pursed
Happiness	Smiling with mouth corners drawn upward, cheeks lifted and a small decrease in distance between eyelids
Surprise	Lifted eyebrows with marked furrows on the forehead, eyes round and mouth open in an oval form
Sadness	Inner part of eyebrows drawn together and narrowing of eyes, wrinkles on forehead and corners of mouth drawn downwards
Anger	Eyebrows drawn downwards and inward, eyes are narrow and staring, forehead smooth, lips pulled tightly, muscles in jaws may be visible
Disgust	Eyebrows drawn downward, upper lip raised and lower lip lowered, nose wrinkled and nasal root widened
Contempt	Mouth corners and eyes lifted, head bent backwards, mouth in scornful grimace
Fear	Eyebrows slightly raised and drawn together with depressed middle part, marked furrows on forehead, eyes wide open with enlarged pupils, mouth open with corners slightly downwards
Shame	Furrows on the forehead, mouth corners pressed together, eyes cast downwards (*NB* Research indicates low recognition agreement)

Based on Izard (1971) and Hjortsjø (1969)

all profit from being able to read facial expressions to identify students' and patients' emotions and predict their thoughts and behaviors in order to assist their learning and coping. The knowledge of this is also useful to the police, who need to identify those who are most likely to respond with violence, as well as to the customs officer who evaluates if it is necessary to do a further search on somebody who seems anxious for some reason.

A more detailed depiction of the main facial expressions of emotions is provided by Fig. 2.1 (see page 10) and Table 2.1. Figure 2.1 shows schematic drawings of facial expressions of seven of the emotions on Izard's list in Table 1.1. The drawings were made by Hjortsjø (1969), who engaged actors to mime the emotions and used these as models for the drawings. Each emotion is shown in a variation of intensity from mild to intense. Table 2.1 includes all emotions in Fig. 2.1, and comprises short descriptions of the characteristic facial features for the emotions on Izard's list except guilt, which has no recognizable facial expression.

There has been much further development of descriptions and pictures, films and videos for coding facial expressions of children as well as adults. A system which has been widely used is Ekman and Friesen's (1975) FACS (Facial Action Coding System), which consists of 44 units related to electronic coding that renders a very comprehensive description of an expression. This, as well as other face-reading soft-ware has been shown to provide quite reliable data for scientific studies.

2.3 What Do Facial Expressions Represent?

Why are emotions expressed openly in facial expressions? Would it not be better if expressions were hidden in ways that each and every one did not have access to one's inner emotions? Most researchers held that it is just the visibility that is the point of the expressions. This is in accordance with Darwin's theory that the function of the facial expression is communication, i.e. that it is used to tell someone of one's experiences of some stimulus, event, or person.

Darwin proposed that emotions can be recognized in purposive behavior, such as in avoiding something to escape from some danger or attack something in order to obtain something to eat. Some behaviors, he held, are evolved as similar for individuals of a species because they have been shown as useful for the species' survival. After being firmly established because of their survival value they are further employed as means of communication.

A series of studies by Susskind et al. (2008) on human faces show support for Darwin's interpretation in the usefulness of facial expressions. The authors found that the communication of fear by wide open eyes and by disgust with compressed eyes due to the downward drawn eyebrows (see Fig. 2.1 and Table 2.1) were associated with, in comparison to a neutral expression, respectively, a larger and a reduced visual field, an increased and a reduced detection of objects, faster and slower eye movements and increased and reduced air respiratory volume. The differences were related to regulation of sensory information that enhances the detection of threat in fear and dampens the unpleasantness of the information in disgust.

Darwin's examples of behaviors in animals which are shown in Fig. 2.2 (see page 12) depict an approaching and threatening dog with bared teeth and one which is submissive and appealing which does not seem to be engaged in goal-oriented behavior. The same is true of the fearful and angry cats. All four seem, rather, to expressing something which "tell" or "communicate" something that might happen or is about to happen.

Darwin held that expressions are almost exclusively used as communication in humans, and that expression and emotion are more or less the same in both animals and man. This can be confirmed, he argued, by the fact that an emotion is more or less intense depending on the intensity of the expression. This means that the emotion is considered as more or less identical to the emotion, i.e. that the expression *is* in fact the emotion, which may be why Darwin did not seem to need a separate definition of emotions.

There is not much disagreement that emotional facial expressions can be a rich and easily accessible source of communication. Most persons will not have problems in using their faces to communicate to someone that an object is attractive,

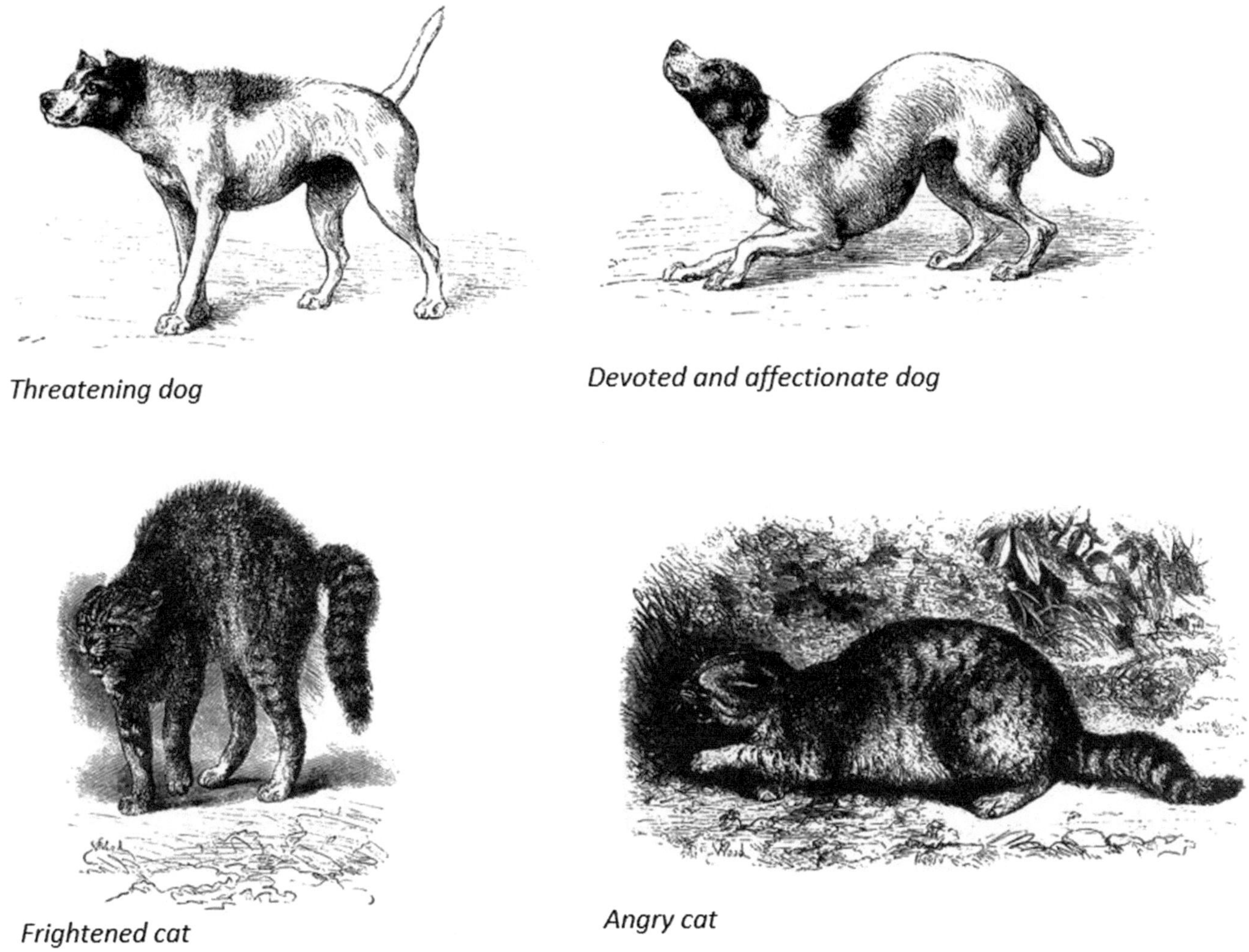

Fig. 2.2 Examples of emotional expressions in animals (from Darwin, 1872)

dangerous or without interest, or that it is good or bad. They will also almost as easily use emotional expressions to communicate relations, such as: «Stay with me», «Come to me», or «Get lost». These are examples of the analog-as distinct from verbal- or digital communication. Analog communication consists of the use of facial expressions as examples or symbols of the message in communication. Thus, it refers to something by being similar to, taking part in, or imitating that which is referred. The dog's bared teeth in Fig. 2.2 form an expression which refers to a rage that implies biting with bared teeth. Another example may be that crying is partaking in the experience of sadness and hurt which is referred to by the facial expression of crying. References of digital, verbal communication are, by contrast, only fortuitously related to that which is referred. Words such as "anger" and "sadness" refers, respectively, to provocative and painful experiences only because of a convention, i.e. because persons agree that this are words which can be employed in certain contexts.

Researchers have proposed that the human face with its scarcity of hair as compared to other animals, and with its layers of muscles to vary the forms of the skin, has been developed in order to increase human's communicative skills. This has been interpreted as the response to a large new need to be able to identify and encode interpersonal signals which emerged when human groups increased in the Pleistocene-period, a period of almost 2 million years for more than 10,000 years ago when the human brain increased three times in size (Baron-Cohen, 1995).

Darwin's view on the close relation between expression and emotion has been especially related to facial expressions in modern theories and research. Izard (1971) held, for instance, that the expression forms a pattern of stimulation on the inside of the face with information to the brain. He assumed, furthermore, that this information, together with information from the body and the senses, leads to the experience of an emotion. The viewpoint can be simplified in a hypothesis that the facial expression causes the emotion, which means, e.g. that you will become happy from smiling and sad from crying. The hypothesis is known as "the facial feedback hypothesis", and has been tested in several studies.

2.4 The Facial Feed-Back Hypothesis

There are different examples of the facial feed-back hypothesis. The most simple and direct type is the proposal that activation of the facial muscles for the expression of an emotion results in information to the brain which leads to the stimulation of an experience of the corresponding emotion.

The hypothesis can be tested by instructing participants without any specific emotion to simulate the expression of an emotion with awareness neither of the emotional significance of the expression nor the fact that the test is related to emotions. The procedure need to include a measure of emotional experience. A very simple and ingenious study along these lines started with instructions to participants that they should read some comic strips and rate the enjoyment of each strips a measure of their emotional experience (Strack, Martin, & Stepper, 1988). Half of the participants in the study were required to hold a pencil with their lips, and the other half to hold a pencil with their teeth when they were reading the comic strips and rating their enjoyment. The point of the procedure is that a pencil held between the teeth provokes a smile, which is a main component of the expression of happiness; whereas a pencil held between the lips have no such effect.

The results were that the participants with artificial smiles because of a pencil between their teeth rated their enjoyment of the comic strips as significantly greater than those who held a pencil between their lips. Enjoyment is an indication of happiness, and the results can, consequently, be considered as support for the feed-back hypothesis.

Duclos et al. (1989) showed that the effect was not limited to positive emotions. The researchers instructed participants who were listening to neutral music to activate facial muscles in ways which produced expressions of fear, anger, disgust and sadness. Emotions were not mentioned in the instructions. Testing consisted of ratings of the intensity of several emotions after the music was stopped. Results supported the feed-back hypothesis by showing higher ratings of the intensity of the emotions which were inadvertently presented by the participants themselves than for other emotions. Several other studies have provided similar support (McIntosh, 1996). A rather original example was an experiment using the neuroxin botulinium («botox»), which paralyzes the facial muscles and is used cosmetically because this hampers the aging process and the development of wrinkles in the face. The results of the experiment were that the injection of botox, which blocks information to the brain, lead to a decreased ability to identify emotions in human faces (Neal & Chartrand, 2011).

Results from studies on several forms of emotional expression indicate that feed-back is not limited to facial stimuli. Persons who have been asked to imitate the bodily carriage characteristic of anger, fear, and sadness have shown higher ratings for the corresponding experiences than for other emotions. Participants in one study were asked to assume the shriveled, forward bent with downcast face bodily carriage typical for depressed persons. The results from the study showed reports of less pride and more negative emotions in these persons than from participants who did not imitate the depressive body. It has also been shown that instructions to talk with a "glad" or a "sad" voice resulted in increases in corresponding ratings of emotional experiences.

Actors are very little surprised by these results. They have, since early in the twentieth century, been practicing "method acting" as taught by the instructor Constantin Stanislavski, who held that the imitation of emotional expressions led to emotional experiences that could be performed in a credible way on the stage. This was a central principle in the education of several of the best-known movie «stars», e.g. Marlon Brando, Marilyn Monroe, Robert de Niro, and Jack Nicholson.

It should be noted, however, that participants in the studies which were cited rated their emotional experiences as "mild". And, furthermore, that stroke patients who have lost their ability of facial expressions (the Mobius syndrome) are nonetheless able to experience emotions. This may suggest that facial expressions may contribute only in part, or may not even be necessary for emotional experiences provided, as is the case with stroke patients, that they have long experience with and have retained the ability to imagine facial expressions.

2.5 Universal Facial Expressions

It was a domineering assumption for many years that facial expressions depended on culture and was, consequently, different from one culture to another. It was ignored or forgotten that Darwin, after receiving responses to questionnaires about children's and adolescents' emotional expressions from missionaries all over the world, concluded that the expressions of several emotions were actually rather similar (see also Chap. 9).

The domineering influence was greatly reduced when Darwin's work was «rediscovered» in the 1960s (see Chap. 11), and new studies related to his findings were designed by Paul Ekman (1973) and Carroll Izard (1971). The most carefully prepared project was carried out by Ekman, and is regarded as a «classical» study in modern research on emotions. Ekman and his co-workers began by inspecting and evaluating around 3000 photos of the faces of adults in order to obtain a representative sample of expressions of various emotions. The photos were all showing white North-Americans, and comprised both spontaneous and posed expressions. Some of the photos were of the researchers themselves, but most of them were selected from diverse sources. A constraint on the selection was that the expression which was shown should correspond to the activation of the corresponding facial muscles.

Ekman's final sample comprised 30 photos of 14 different persons, and referred to six photos of each of the emotions happiness, sadness, anger, fear, surprise, and disgust. Participants from five different countries were shown the photos and were tested for their identification of the emotion on each photo by pointing to a list of words for different emotions. Examples of photos and results from Ekman's study are shown in Fig. 2.3 (see page 15). The numbers in the figure represent percentage of agreement about the emotions shown in photos of facial expressions of emotions among respondents from each of the five countries. Figure 2.3 shows, for instance, that 97% of U.S participants and 95% of Brazilians agreed that photos of happiness pertained to happiness, that 68% of Chileans and 85% of U.S participants agreed that fear photos showed fear, and that 90% of the Japanese and 92% of the Argentinians have agreed that the photos of disgusting facial expressions pertained to disgust.

The results can generally be interpreted as showing a high degree of agreement about the facial expression of the six emotions which were entered in the study. Ekman pointed out that the results pertained to persons from four different languages (English, Japanese, Portuguese, and Spanish) and from three cultural groups (Anglo-American, Latin-American, and Japanese). The results from Izard's study showed similar levels of agreement for the same emotions as Ekman's among participants from European countries (England, France, Germany, Greece, Sweden, and Switzerland). Agreement was, however, much lower for shame than for the other emotions, and lower among participants from Japan and Africa. The latter seemed to be due to the fact that these participants were the only ones who were not tested in their natural language.

The results show some variation in agreement for different emotions. Both Ekman's and Izard's study showed highest agreement for happiness, surprise, and disgust, and somewhat lower for fear and anger. This can be due to several factors. The photos for some of the emotions may, for example, have been slightly clearer or more characteristic of the emotion in question than others. It can also be assumed that the results were affected, as was noted by Ekman, by cultural variation in language and the frequency of emotional expression in a country or culture. Anger, which showed the lowest percentage for Japan in Fig. 2.3, is for instance very controlled and seldom shown openly in Japanese culture. Infrequent experience with expressions of an emotion may result in insecure identification of a pictured emotion, and in lower agreement about these pictures both within a across cultural groups.

Criticisms of Ekman's studies were mainly directed at Ekman's method. A central objection was that agreement among participants was inflated by the use of a list of words where only one of them pertained directly to the photograph (Russell, 1994). This argument is countered by the fact that the participants in Izard's (1971) study, which yielded similar results to Ekman's, responded by using free descriptions of the expressions, as well as by alternative methods with variations in the contents of the response lists. Subsequent research has generally been supportive for Ekman's results, but has also confirmed that there may be some cultural variation in recognition (or clarity) of facial expressions. It has, for example, been shown that agreement on facial expressions for pictures of persons within a culture is larger than for pictures of persons from another culture.

It may be noted as a summary of this research that studies of recognition of facial expressions have provided stable evidence that the expressions have a universal form, at least for the emotions which were employed in Ekman's study. This has been interpreted by Ekman and Izard, following Darwin, to mean that the facial expression mirrors a human "nature" which is hardwired and coded in a neurological program. Indications of universality are often used in this way to support biological explanations and to conceive of emotions as basic, but this is weakened by the fact that social emotions do not show universal facial expressions. It should also be noted that the studies pertain to facial expressions and not to emotions. Studies on the recognition of emotions should need to include indications of typical contexts and/or scenes in addition to depiction of facial expressions (see Sect. 9.3).

2.6 Facial Expressions as Subcortical Stimulation: Dimberg, Thunberg, & Elmehed's (2000) Study

The face and its expression are, as was hinted at in Sect. 2.1, not any stimulus. It is among other things also a stimulus which seems to trigger imitation. Meltzoff and Moore (1983, 1989) showed in a series of well-known studies that newborns imitated another person's facial changes, such as opening and closing of the mouth and protrusion of the tongue. As this imitation is scarcely based on conscious experience by the newborn, it can be assumed that it related to the subcortical structures which were the basis for responses in Øhman and Soares' (1994) study cited in Sect. 1.7.

The significance of a subcortical imitation of facial expression is that this may mediate an "infection" of emotion from one person to another by facial feed-back. This is further discussed in Sect. 4.6. A study directly related to the emotional response to subcortically presented stimulation has been conducted Dimberg, Thunberg, and Elmehed (2000). The study comprised three groups of students as participants. The procedure started with participants (individually) in front of a PC which showed enlarged photos of a neutral face for a first group of participants, a face with an angry expression for a second group, and a face with a happy expression for the third group. The photos were shown in 30 ms and were either presented openly (the neutral photo) or were immediately followed (photos of angry or happy expressions) by neutral photos in 100 ms according to the backward masking method (see Sect. 1.7). The participants were, consequently, not able to be aware of or to remember the emotional expressions. Responses were measured in terms of miniature electrodes on the facial muscles zygomatic major and corrugator supercilii, which are active in, respectively, the facial expressions of happiness and anger. This measurement is known as electromyography (EMG).

The results from the study indicated a more vigorous arousal in the "angry" corrugator than in the "happy" zygomatic, but the main point was that the "happy" zygomatic was clearly more strongly activated by presentation of the happy than by the angry stimulus face, whereas the "angry" corrugator showed

Fig. 2.3 Percentage agreement in how photographs were judged across cultures (from Ekman, 1973)

	Percentage Agreement in How Photograph Was Judged Across Cultures				
	United States (*N*=99)	Brazil (*N*=40)	Chile (*N*=119)	Argentina (*N*=168)	Japan (*N*=29)
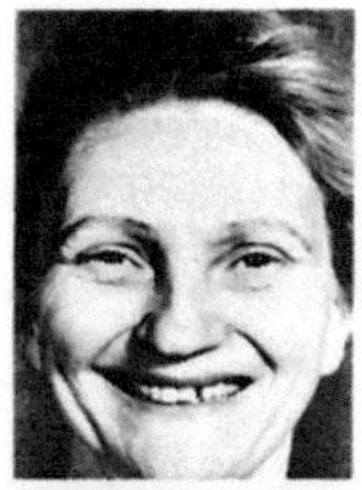	97% Happiness	95% Happiness	95% Happiness	98% Happiness	100% Happiness
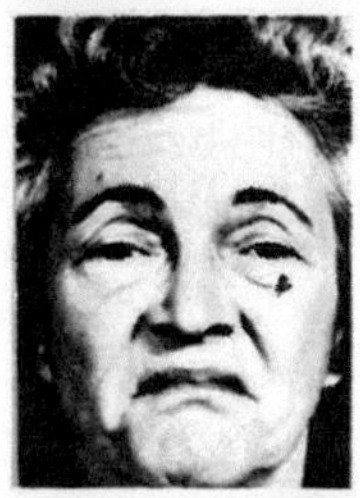	92% Disgust	97% Disgust	92% Disgust	92% Disgust	90% Disgust
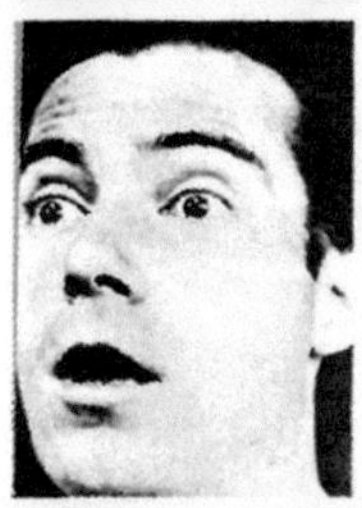	95% Surprise	87% Surprise	93% Surprise	95% Surprise	100% Surprise
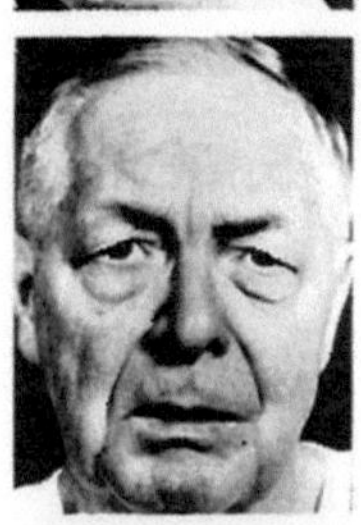	84% Sadness	59% Sadness	88% Sadness	78% Sadness	62% Sadness
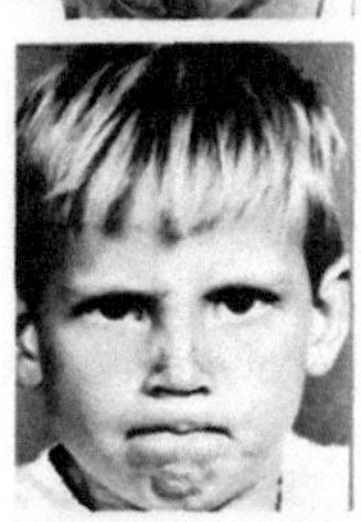	67% Anger	90% Anger	94% Anger	90% Anger	90% Anger
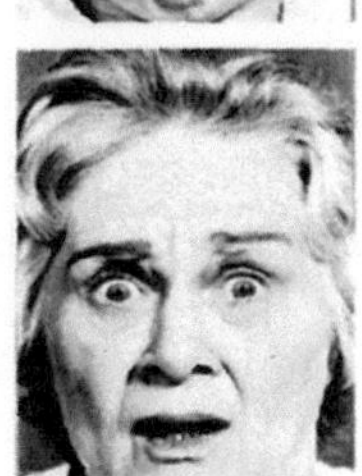	85% Fear	67% Fear	68% Fear	54% Fear	66% Fear

the opposite low activation of the happy and much stronger activation after the angry face. Or, in other words, a happy face triggered a response in perceivers' "happy-" and an angry face triggered a response in their "angry" muscle.

Dimberg et al.'s study showed, then, that there was muscular activity in participants' faces corresponding to emotional expressions in another face which they were not aware of. This can be interpreted as an unconscious, emotional imitation where the emotional expression in one person's face may evoke some resonance through facial feed-back in another. This is a subcortical imitation that shows a parallel to conceptions in modern neuroscience that humans participate in each other's neural networks. A basis for this concept is the discovery of "mirror neurons", i.e. neurons which are activated in the same area of the brain in a seated person as the neuronal activation in a person who is observed by the seated person to perform some active task. The seated person's neuronal activation in this instance can be said to mirror the neuronal activation of the active person. Mirror neurons were originally discovered in apes by researchers in Parma in Italy (Rizzolatti, Fadiga, Gallese, & Fandassi, 1996), and have been shown in humans by a large number of studies, including studies of muscular activity in the face (Enticott et al., 2008). The neurons have been interpreted by researchers as examples that humans participate and share each other's experiences (Gallese, 2003, 2011), but there is some controversy whether this extends to the emotions (Decety, 2010).

2.7 Practical Relevance

Facial expressions are directly related to communication on different levels. It can stimulate improved communication on the personal level by providing a standard for practice both in recognition of emotions in others and in heightening one's own consciousness as regards one's communication of emotions to others. Group practice with miming is often an enjoyable as well as a useful experience in this context. The identification of the main muscles of the face may serve as useful cues. On the level of official and electronic communication there is a large and underdeveloped potential to use easily identifiable facial expressions as indicators that can clarify and/or reinforce verbal directions and explanations which are often long, abstract and complicated. Facial expressions are used as an analog language long before children learn to speak (see Chap. 5), which also suggests a level of international, or global communication where communicative doors may be opened with the use of the facial language.

There is a large application based on the detailed descriptions of facial muscles as regards identification and treatment of human problems. Examples are that patients with Huntington's illness have been shown to have problems in identifying negative emotions, especially anger, that patients with Parkinson's illness have problems in identifying sadness and fear, that patients with Alzheimer's disorder have problems in identifying sadness, and that persons with Asperger's syndrome show a general problem in recognizing all basic emotions. Studies have also shown large problems in identification of emotions in persons with schizophrenia, obsessive-compulsive disorder and depression.

2.8 Summary

The face is a primary arousal of attention and a center of the expression of many, perhaps most of the emotions. Variations in expressions are based on the activation of two levels of muscles that are activated separately to form the skin in different ways.

Darwin noted similarities in expression of emotions in animals and man and conceived of a very close relation between the expression and the emotion. He also held that the expression was based on inherited circuits in the brain, and that the expression functions mainly as communication in humans.

Tests for the relation between facial expression and emotional experience, which has been stated as a feed-back hypothesis, have shown that simulation or imitation of the facial expression of an emotion may lead to experiences of the corresponding emotion.

Darwin's concepts of the universality of emotional expression has been rediscovered and tested by several researchers. The main study was conducted by Ekman, and showed, in support of Darwin, a high degree of agreement about the facial expressions for happiness, surprise, anger, sadness, fear, and disgust among participants from different languages and cultures.

Observations of newborns' imitation of facial characteristics lead to the assumption that emotional facial expressions may be imitated (and infected) at a subcortical level. The feasibility of this conception was demonstrated in Dimberg et al's study, which showed that observer's emotional facial muscles were activated by photos of emotional facial expressions which the observers could not be consciously aware of. This unconscious imitation may be a parallel phenomenon to mirror neurons.

Reflection Questions

1. What would be the consequences if you and/or your closest persons were: (a) Able to control your facial expressions perfectly? (b) Were without any variations in facial expressions whatsoever?
2. What may be consequences of people's subconscious emotional responses to other person's facial expressions? Could they be limited to only a few emotions?

Research/Exercise Examples

1. Find descriptions of facial muscles on the net which can be used to identify the facial muscles zygomatic and corrugator in your own and your study colleagues' faces.
2. Facial expressions which are universal and inherited should be immediately accessible for imitation. Test this assumption by recording the time it will take a participant in a study-group to imitate an emotion on request.

3. Test your reading of facial expressions by positing yourself at a place where you can watch persons passing. Note for each person if you can identify a specific emotion and your confidence (insecure—moderately secure—very secure) in the identification. Note also the sex and approximate age (child, adolescent, young adult, older adult) of the person. To what extent do you think the results reflect your ability to identify, the accessibility of facial expressions or the subject (type of person)?

Further Reading

Dimberg, U., Thunberg, M., & Elmehed, K. (2000). Unconscious facial reactions to emotional facial expressions. *Psychological Science, 11*, 86–89.

Ekman, P. (1973). Cross-cultural studies of facial expression. In P. Ekman (Ed.), *Darwin and facial expression* (pp. 169–222). New York: Academic Press.

Niedenthal, P. M., Krauth-Gruber, S., & Ric, F. (2006). *Psychology of emotion* (pp. 115–154). New York: Psychology Press.

Individual Emotions

3

A main theme of the two first chapters was that emotions consist of different types. This is extended in this chapter by descriptions of functions, experiences, causes and consequences for each of the ten emotions on Izard's list, as well as for pride, envy, and jealousy, which seem to be present in all known cultures. 11 of the emotions are assumed to include a core relational theme, which refers to the meaning in terms of the harm or benefit for relationships implied in an emotion (Lazarus, 1991).

Emotions can be experienced and expressed in a variation of intensity. It is, for instance, a large difference between being angry and mad and between being afraid and scared stiff. These differences cannot be described in the overviews in the present chapter, and the presentation refers, consequently, to the normal type of each emotion.

The chapter includes results from studies where experiences of emotions were tested for their meaning by rating scales for participants' evaluation of the extent to which each emotion was experienced as pleasant, tense (in terms arousal), controlled and supportive of self-esteem (Izard, 1991). Note that control is the opposite of impulsivity, and that low control therefore means high impulsivity. This chapter also includes research on persons' awareness of physiological signals of individual emotions.

3.1 Positive Emotions: Happiness, Interest, and Surprise

Positive emotions are historically ignored in research, but a marked increase in interest has been evident the last 10–15 years. An example is Fredrickson's (1998, 2001) theory about positive emotions' functioning to broaden and build the adaptation. «Broaden» refers to the openness to new perspectives, challenges, and learning which can be the effects of attention, thinking and behavior. Happiness leads, for instance, to a creative and flexible testing in play, interest leads to exploration and examination, and pride to the sharing of positive attainments with others. A support for this is that positive emotions can be associated with open, flexible, and creative solutions to problems (see Chap. 6).

«Building» in Fredrickson's theory refers to stimulation of consistency and duration, i.e. that one continues the play and interested examination which is implied in positive emotions. This continuity is related to the survival of the human species. Humans are dependent on others in many years before the can be independent actors, and they need therefore a long period of stability and continuity to build their learning and experience.

3.1.1 Happiness

Function. Happiness is central in social interaction which leads to the establishment and strengthening of relationships and participation in the community. The emotion leads to a relaxed, open behavioral attitude which communicates good intentions, openness and space for social interaction. This leads to mutual trust, which opens up for personal conversations and close contacts. The core theme for happiness is progress towards personal goals.

Experience. The experience of happiness has been described as well-being, lightness, release, pleasantness, relaxation and delight. The experience may also show elements of meaningfulness, safety, and trustfulness and a tendency to be open, inviting and supportive in relation to others. Ratings of meaning suggest that happiness is conceived as a pleasant emotion which triggers little tension, do not show much need of control and is positive for self-esteem. Physiological signals for happiness have been noted as the feelings of warm and relaxed muscles, changes in the voice and much verbalization (talk).

Causes and consequences. The most frequent causes of happiness are, according to research results, to engender happiness in the family and in other close persons, the perception of love in one's closest persons, and the ability to share time, experiences and emotions with them. Other causes are being with friends, success in difficult tasks and the experience that one has many possibilities (Bartlett & Izard, 1972). Happiness leads to an open, playful and creative manner. This may result in some superficiality in terms of a simplified manner of thinking and an overestimation of one's own competence. The emotion leads, furthermore, to a reduction in tension and relaxation of muscles which improves blood flow and may be preventive of health problems.

A. Vikan, *A Fast Road to the Study of Emotions*,
DOI 10.1007/978-3-319-52313-2_3

3.1.2 Interest

Function. Interest leads to learning, increased knowledge and building of experience. This means that interest is a driver of cognition (attention, memory, and thinking), which is the reason that researchers have pointed to interest as the most basic of the emotions (Frijda, 2007; Izard, 2007, 2009). There is, however, no defined core theme for interest.

Experience. Interest comprises experiences of being awake and in control, and being concentrated and engaged in something which is meaningful. Interest is, like happiness, associated with a high degree of pleasure and as a support of a persons' positive self-esteem, i.e. her-his emotional attitude toward him-herself (see Sect. 4.4), but is held to imply a higher degree of tension and challenge to control. There is noted no specific experiences of physiological signals related to interest.

Causes and consequences. Interest is activated by stimulation which is new, unexpected and interesting and includes images, thoughts and memories. It leads to a focus and concentration on a subject or an area, and is followed up by new experiences over time. This leads to a continuity in projects and plans that keeps a person in interaction with the surroundings and serves to strengthen the adaptation by adding information and establishing overviews and realistic control.

3.1.3 Surprise

Function. The function of surprise is to prepare to explore something by pausing to collecting one's thoughts in order to identify the cause of the surprise. There has not been defined a core theme for surprise.

Experience. The experience is described as being shaken, shocked and wide awake. This is sometimes blended with feelings of confusion, embarrassment and being lost. Surprise makes persons stop and be mentally "empty" before they experience a sudden incident as breach with their expectations or as something which is outside of what they had imagined. Ratings of meaning for surprise were parallel to happiness and interest for pleasure and self-esteem, and were more similar to happiness than interest for tension and control. Surprise has not been associated with specific physiological signals.

Causes and consequences. The cause of surprise is a clearly marked incidence or event which happens suddenly and unexpectedly. Surprise leads to a break in ongoing activities in order to address the sudden and new challenge, and may result in new experiences and learning which serves as an initial phase of interest.

3.2 Negative Emotions: Sadness, Anger, Disgust, Contempt, Shame and Guilt

Negative emotions lead to a narrowing in focus on causes, and a tendency of avoidance or termination of the discomfort usually associated with the experience of these emotions. Research has been focused much more frequently on negative than positive emotions. The prime reason for this is that the negative emotions often are problems both to individuals and society. This is shown in sadness (in terms of depression), and fear (in terms of anxiety) which are part of the symptoms of many types of mental disorder, while anger (in terms of aggression) is the main content in social problems (war, criminality). Negative emotions, especially fear and anger, have in addition been focused because they can easily be defined behaviorally and be systematically explored in experimentation with animals.

3.2.1 Sadness

Function. The function of sadness is to seek or to attract help and support. This reinforces social contact and interaction. Sadness, furthermore, reinforces attachments because it is often related to lack and loss of persons which underlines their significance in persons' lives. The core theme for sadness has been defined, accordingly, as irreparable loss.

Experience. Sadness is generally an experience of being heavy. The limbs and the body are experienced as heavy, mental processes such as thinking and remembering are experienced as heavy and the very being in the world is tinted with the experience of heavy. The sadness experience may also include a mental pain in the breast which is felt as a pressure. Other aspects of the experience are loneliness, loss of contact with others and an experience of having been betrayed and deserted by others. Sad persons often conceive of themselves as small and unsuccessful, as weak and closed and little attractive to others, and with impulses to withdraw from the outside world (Lambie & Marcel, 2002).

Ratings of the meaning of sadness suggest that the emotion is little pleasant, implies a weakening of self-esteem and is associated with high tension and little possibility of control. Physiological signals have been noted as lumps in the throat, pressure on the breast and an unruly stomach.

Causes and consequences. The most frequent causes of sadness are loss of and/or separation from close others in terms of death, divorce or a long journey. Other causes are rejection, betrayal and disappointment in others and failure of obtaining one's goals. The general consequences are passivity and withdrawal from others together with thoughts that one may not pester others with one's negative experiences and problems.

3.2.2 Anger

Function. The function of anger is to guard against threats and to fight obstacles. Core theme is to limit and/or oppose persons, events or forces directed against the person her/himself and/or the closest persons.

Experience. Anger is initially experienced as being impeded and suppressed by someone or something. This is followed by experiences of being insulted and violated and by a wish to attack. The experience of the expression of anger is dominated by an experience of mobilization of muscles in the limbs. This frequently entails an experience of warmth which relates to experiences of initiative, courage, bravery and strength which may seem just and liberating. Additional experiences are impulses to use aggression to remove hindrances, and wishes to hurt and damage someone or something.

The meaning with anger is rated in ways which show a picture of a somewhat self-contradictory, high tension emotion which may not be very pleasurable but may increase self-esteem even though is implies little possibility of control. Anger has been associated with physiological signals such as strenuous breathing, feelings of coldness and shivering together with warmness in the cheeks, a more rapid frequency in heart beats, tense muscles and changes in the voice.

Causes and consequences. The common causes of anger are aggression from others, unfair treatment, being fooled or harassed in some way, or being hindered from something one wants to do or to obtain. The best known consequences of anger are behaviors that hurt and/or violate other persons in ways that are frequent in criminal acts, conflicts and war. This may lead to revenge and to retaliations which can form a destructive circle. What is often overlooked is that anger may imply positive consequences such as honesty and sincerity, and that the emotion is useful and at times necessary in order to remove distracting obstacles to accomplish a task.

3.2.3 Fear

Function: Fear is very clearly related to survival by being primarily aimed at avoiding danger by hiding, immobilization, or flight. Core theme is to be confronted with a concrete and overwhelming danger.

Experience: It is typical of the experience of fear to feel threatened, in danger, vulnerable, alone, lost, and isolated. Fear also implies experiences of insecurity and of being overwhelmed and in the process of being destroyed. Ratings of meaning indicate that fear is associated with a low degree of pleasure, a decrease in self-esteem, very high tension and a low possibility of control. Fear is the emotion which, together with happiness and anger, shows the highest number of physiological signals. These are strenuous breath, unruly stomach, experiences of coldness and sweating on the skin, and rapid heart-beats.

Causes and consequences: Causes of fear are perils such as floods, landslides, strokes of lightening, dangerous animals, high-speed cars and hostile persons. The central consequence of fear is a mobilization where energy is transferred from the digestion to the muscles and is experienced in terms of physiological signals. This may also include a sharpening of the senses to discover danger which may result in headache and lower tolerance for bright light and high sounds.

3.2.4 Disgust

Function: The function of disgust is to protect against pollution which may result in contamination and/or to contact with parasites. Core theme is aversion against accepting or being near an indigestible object or, metaphorically, a person, an idea or a viewpoint.

Experience: The experience of disgust is characterized by aversion and avoidance. This relates especially to taking something in the mouth, but the experience is also related to smell, touch, and visual perception. The aversion may stimulate the stomach to heave and to a need to throw up. The heaving sensation is the only physiological signal of disgust. Disgust has not been rated for meaning.

Causes and consequences: The main cause is held to be biologically based and is the smell which suggests rotten food or polluted drink. This is assumed to generalize to smell and touch related to feces and sexuality. Disgust motivates to care in selection, storing and preparation of food as well as care with personal hygiene (Rozin, Lowry, Imada, & Haidt, 1999; Rozin, Haidth, & McCauley, 2008).

3.2.5 Contempt

Function: The function of contempt is assumed to be to decrease fear of an enemy and to stimulate initiative in preparation for aggression/battle. There is not defined a core theme for contempt.

Experience: The experience of contempt is dominated by a feeling of superiority, especially in relation to winning a competition. This is especially salient and stimulated in a person who has felt underestimated and opposed, and triumphing shows very clear marks of contempt. Izard (1991) referred to results from a study which showed that contempt was the «cold» emotion in a hostile triad of anger, disgust and contempt. The emotion has not been rated for meaning, and has not been conceived as associated with physiological signals.

Causes and consequences: There is no study of the causes of contempt, but it has been assumed that the emotion may serve as a defense against feelings of insecurity and/or lack of competence. Contempt is a problematic emotion because it may easily be part of discriminations of individuals and groups of persons.

3.2.6 Shame

Function: The function of shame is to reduce tendencies toward self-assertion and narcissism. This serves to avoid that individuals demand unjust parts of means which are distributed among groups of persons and society. Core theme for shame is to fail to live up to one's own standards and ideals. Shame is the only emotion which has been assumed as domineering for the formation of whole cultures (Abu-Lughod, 1986; Benedict, 1946; Peristiany, 1974).

Experience: The experience of shame is described generally as a painfully negative experience of oneself. A shameful person experiences her/himself as incompetent and without value, laughable, weak and little attractive. The shame experience is also related to experiences of being rejected, defenseless, clumsy and with low intelligence, as well as to experiences of oneself as a looser, being exposed to others perception and to wishes to shrink or sink into the earth. Rating of the meaning of shame shows that shame implies little pleasure, weakening of self-esteem, high degree of tension and a middle-range possibility to gain control. Physiological signals have been registered as sweating, warmth in the cheeks and increase in heart-beat frequency.

Causes and consequences: Shame is especially aroused by rejections and/or by not succeeding in relation to important other persons. The consequences may be to attack or to withdraw totally. The source of shameful experiences is held to be the person her/himself rather than a specific behavior. Shame is, therefore, more difficult to regulate than other emotions, such as for instance guilt. This is because the object of regulation in shame is the person him/herself, whereas the object in guilt is some behavior. Regulations of oneself has no clear object, which may be the reason that self-regulation of shame in Japanese culture is ritual suicide (seppuku). The regulation of guilt may on the other hand be related to a specific behavior in terms of promises to stop or change the behavior, ask for forgiveness or pay for negative consequences.

3.2.7 Guilt

Function: The function of guilt is to regulate behavior in conformity to ethical norms. Core theme is the violation of a moral rule.

Experience: The experience of guilt is characterized by the experience of having done something wrong or by not having done something right. The experience comprises repetitious thoughts and remorse related to this, as well as acceptance of being responsible for or causing the negative incident. Ratings of the meaning of guilt are similar to those for shame by showing low pleasure, weakening of self-esteem, high degree of tension and some, but not as large possibility of control. Guilt is well known for physiological signals, but results from studies have not identified specific responses.

Causes and consequences: The cause of guilt is, as was indicated in the description of experiences, thoughts that one has caused or been responsible for a morally wrong behavior or incidence. The consequences are mainly the repetitious rumination about the incidence. This entails thoughts about what might have been different, what might have happened if events unfolded in other ways, etc.

3.3 Other Emotions: Pride, Envy, and Jealousy

Pride, envy, and jealousy are recognized in the literature as salient determinants of human behavior. Anthropological descriptions suggest that they are present in people in all cultures, and it might well be assumed that they are part of our common human ancestry. It is therefore a little strange that these emotions have almost been ignored in research. There is little information on facial characteristics, meaning and physiological signals related to these emotions.

3.3.1 Pride

Function: The function of pride has been envisaged as support for the development of activities and learning. The reason for this is that pride yields confidence in oneself and a push which is useful in interaction with others. Core theme for pride has been described as an augmentation of ego-identity by attributing the cause of a valuable creation or obtainment to the effort of oneself or to one's group.

Experience: The experience of pride may be differentiated as «authentic pride» and "hubris". Authentic pride is an experience of satisfaction and delight related to one's own achievement. This is a pride which is naturally associated with experiences of mastery, development and competence. Hubris represents, on the other hand, an overvaluing of one's own significance, competencies and possibilities which are represented as arrogance, conceit, and/or inflatedness (Tracy & Robins, 2007).

Causes and consequences: The most direct cause of pride is to succeed as expected or above expectations. The consequences of the emotion are different for the two types. Authentic pride results in a self-confidence which also is positive for a person's relationships. Hubris is a form of narcissism which is associated with devaluation and/or open aggression towards others.

3.3.2 Envy

Function: Evolutionary psychologists have proposed that the function of envy in a world with limited resources is to note that one has been distanced by competing others and to act accordingly (Hill & Buss, 2008). Core theme for envy was proposed as a wish to have something that belongs to others and associated to a conception of justice (Smith, 1991).

Experience: The experience of envy is the wish for another person's qualities, belongings or skills which are experienced as better than one's own. The wish is not that one should necessarily obtain something from the other, but that the other has something which is perceived as better. This can be experienced as unacceptable and almost unbearable. The emotion is not aroused when the envied other's qualities and objects are no longer in existence (Schoeck, 1969). A study of several hundred persons' experience of envy showed that the salient themes were longing for something that were owned or controlled by another or by others, experiences of inferiority associated with sadness, anxiety, anger and bitterness against the other, or others, which were perceived as causes of the emotion.

Causes and consequences: The cause of envy is inherent in the characterization of the experience, and comprises specifically the experience of being or having less than others. The consequences of envy seem to be most salient in relation to close and envied persons who seem similar to oneself. Envy is therefore not primarily a response to social inequalities. The consequences are related to the fact that envy resonances or mirrors the person as inferior to others. This is shown to result in experiences of inferiority, sadness, and helplessness, but this may also arouse intense hostility and aggression (Leach, 2008; Smith & Kim, 2007).

3.3.3 Jealousy

Function: The function of jealousy is not very clear. Hupka (1991) proposed that jealousy may have a different function for women and men. He held that jealousy is useful for women because it can serve to hinder that the partner uses resources on others than on the shared children. Men's envy was held to be useful because it may hinder that energy is wasted in raising other person's children. Core theme for jealousy has been proposed as a perceived violation that a third party has caused loss or threats of loss of reciprocal love from a loved other person.

Experience: The experience of jealousy comprises an anxiety to lose an important relationship to another person. This implies that others are considered as more important and may be preferred to oneself. Jealousy was evaluated as more intense than envy, and as high on measures of distrust, fear, insecurity, and loneliness in a study by Parrott and Smith (1993). Results from interviews have suggested that the experience of jealousy is characterized by an anxious insecurity related to the possibility of losing someone, blended with feelings of hurt, sadness and suspiciousness of betrayal. It has also been suggested that the experience of jealousy vary dependent on whether it relates to a suspicion of something, or to an actual infidelity or a broken relationship, which may result in, respectively, a «suspicious» or a "reactive jealousy" (Bringle, 1991). The suspicious form is characterized by vigilance, uneasiness and worry, and the reactive form by anger, sadness and fear of the future. See also Hart and Legerstee (2010).

Causes and consequences: The causes of jealousy is the experience that an important relationship to another person is about to be lost and taken over by a third party. The descriptions of the experience show that jealousy is a deep and inclusive experience. The consequences of this may be extensive and include loss of concentration and rumination which may result in problems at work or with studies. The consequences also include phantasies about the other persons which are involved included in the jealousy. This leads easily to anger and to wishes to confront the other and to revenge which may end in violence.

3.4 Practical Relevance

The content of the experience of individual emotions may contribute to a more extensive insight into the implications of each of them. It should be noticed that different functions lead to very different behaviors, which is one of the main points of the characteristics of selective drivers (Sect. 1.5). It is important to be aware of this because different emotions are often aroused either at the same time or a short time after each other (see Sect. 13.1). The problem in these situations is that different emotions instigate different behaviors and it is difficult to know one's own emotions as well as to react adequately. An overview of the emotions and a process toward coping may best be started by making an inventory of the emotions which are involved, the causes of each of them and the behaviors which they suggest.

The main message in this chapter is that each emotion has individual characteristics. This should form a background for a skeptical attitude toward general proposals about emotions, such as "emotions are destructive to reason" and "emotions are neurologically based on the amygdala". General proposals such as these are weakened by, respectively, evidence in Chap. 6 that the effect of emotion on cognition is markedly different for happiness and sadness, and evidence in Chap. 12 that amygdala is the neurological center for fear, but not for disgust.

Teil I

Table 3.1 Key terms for functions, experiences and causes of 13 emotions

Emotion	*Function*	*Characteristics of experience*	*Central cause*
Happiness	Establish social contact	Well-being, lightness, relaxation	Making others happy
Interest	Learning, building experience	Being awake and concentrated	Interesting news
Surprise	Prepare exploration	Being shaken and awake	Sudden and un-expected incidence
Sadness	Strengthen social relationships	Feeling heavy loss, pain	Loss, separation
Anger	Defense against threat	Being violated, arousal	Injustice, being hindered
Fear	Avoid danger	Threatened, vulnerable, alone	Physical danger
Disgust	Protect against pollution	Aversion and disgust	Bad smell from food and drink
Contempt	Decrease fear of an enemy	Superiority	Defense against insecurity
Shame	Reduction of self-assertion	Worthless, laughable, weak	Rejection, failure
Guilt	Complying with norms	Did a moral wrong, remorse	Cause of some moral wrong
Pride	Support for activity and learning	Satisfaction and happiness over achievements	Success at something
Envy	Defense against losing a competition	Wishes for other person's qualities and/or belongings	Experience of being or having less than another
Jealousy	Unclear	Fear of losing the relationship to another person	Experience of threat to a relationship

3.5 Summary

A summary of this chapter is shown in Table 3.1.

Reflection Questions

1. Individual emotions are often considered as qualitative types. Which qualities (e.g. color, mobility, clearness, directionality, attraction) do you associate to interest, happiness, anger, fear, envy, and jealousy?
2. In what way have happiness and interest served to broaden and build your personal life?

Research/Exercise Examples

1. The lack of universal facial expressions of shame, pride, envy, and jealousy do not mean that they are not easily recognized. Test this by covertly assigning two of these emotions to each student in your group and having them enacted and guessed at in front of the others. Note that recognition is shown both in enactment and guessing.
2. The descriptions of functions related to individual emotions are mainly influenced by evolutionary theory, but do they agree with people's own views? This can be tested by asking persons to what extent on a five-point scale of not at all—a little—some—much—very much they think that being (interested, happy, angry, sad, etc. …) make them: (a) be more popular with others, (b) become more efficient in work, (c) avoid others, (d) be a less considerate person, (e) be more creative. NB: You should probably not ask each person for more than five emotions.

Further Reading

Izard, C. E. (1991). *The psychology of emotions*. New York: Plenum Press.

Lewis, M. (2008). Self-Conscious emotions: Embarassment, pride, shame, and guilt. In M. Lewis, J. M. Haviland-Jones & L. Feldman Barrett (Eds.), *Handbook of emotions. Third Edition* (pp. 742–756). New York: Guilford.

Power, M., & Dalgleish, T. (1997). *Cognition and emotion* (pp. 197–439). East Sussex, UK: Psychology Press.

Personal Indications

4

The aim of the three first chapters was to describe the general characteristics of emotions. This may have resulted in a relative ignorance of the fact that emotions are experienced as intimate and subjective and characteristic of a person. Chapter 3 provided some cues to how emotions are central to the experience. This is further discussed at the start of this chapter by reference to the experience of emotions as directly related at and transforming reality, which leads to variations in the intensity and how this is related to behavior and adaptation. It is noted that emotional experiences resonates with persons' self and can be internalized in their personality, and that this, in addition to their relation to adaptation, may serve as a source of fear. The last part of the chapter comprise a further presentation of evidence that emotions may be contagious, and a discussion on results from studies which shows that the experience of emotions results in a need for social sharing.

4.1 The Experience of Emotion: Emotions as Truth

Studies of emotional experiences have been conducted by phenomenological descriptions in two different ways. A phenomenological description is an attempt to characterize the remarkable and fundamental characteristics of the experience. This has led to a characterization of emotional experience as *directed at* something, as *transforming* that which it is directed at and to imply a *lack of self-consciousness* (Lambie & Marcel, 2002). *Directed at* something means that emotional experience is *about and concerns* something, it is not an experience *of* something. The experience *transforms* that which it is directed at by attaching an emotional quality to the experience. Fear has, for instance attached the quality of "threatening", which transforms the experience of the world as something which is dangerous, while happiness has attached the quality of "attractive", which transforms the experience of the world as engaging, pleasant and likable (see also Sect. 1.5).

An *experience without self-consciousness* means that emotional experience is an experience that something exists in a certain way, in contradistinction to the experience of something as being an experience of this or that. An example may be that when you are happy for something you experience things and events as positive and as being or existing in that way. You do not experience your happiness as an experience or perception *of* something rather than the thing itself. The happiness is, in other words, taken to refer to the world rather than to the experience of the world. This implies that emotions are experiences that something is valid and true. The experience of fear leads for instance to an experience that something is dangerous, and means that when you fear something the feared object is experienced as being dangerous. Thus, the logic of the emotional experience transforms the world into an experiential truth. This experience is reinforced by the fact that emotions are seldom initiated by oneself but as something which happens to us. The attribution of truth, furthermore, increases as the intensity of the experience increases, and a very intense positive emotion may lead to an experience which is felt as a revelation.

One of the methods in doing research on the experiences of emotions has been conducted by standardized interviews or questionnaires about characteristics and contexts related to the arousal and maintenance of one specific or several emotions. The main disadvantage with this method is that responses refer to memories rather than to direct experiences of emotions. It is also a drawback that reasoning related to the question, for instance: "How long did your anger last"? may interfere with the experience itself. One of the most reliable and valid method is probably the use of diaries. An example is Oatley and Duncan's (1992) study where students use diaries to enter, each night in a period of several weeks, the frequency, intensity, content and cause of their emotions during the same day. The results showed (e.g.) that the content of their experiences were noted as thoughts in 81% of the entries, as changes in their bodies in 77%, and as a readiness to act in 90%. Note that this mirrors our definition of emotions in Sect. 1.1.

The other type of method can be combined with the former, and consists of ratings of emotions in relation to dimensions of the experience. Results from a study comprising rating of the experiences of eight emotions in four dimensions were cited in Chap. 3. Table 4.1 (see page 26) provides an example of this study by showing the three items for rating experiences on the dimensions of tension and control (impulsivity). The instruction was that participants should imagine a typical situation of

A. Vikan, *A Fast Road to the Study of Emotions*,
DOI 10.1007/978-3-319-52313-2_4

Teil I

Table 4.1 Examples of rating items for the tension and control dimensions in Bartlett-Izard's dimensional rating

Instruction: Imagine a situation pertaining to happiness, and mark the rating alternative which shows your opinion							
	Not at all		Moderately		Extremely		
How tense do you feel?	0	1	2	3	4	5	6
How tense are your thoughts?	0	1	2	3	4	5	6
How tense is your behavior?	0	1	2	3	4	5	6
How impulsive do you feel?	0	1	2	3	4	5	6
How impulsive are your thoughts?	0	1	2	3	4	5	6
How impulsive is your behavior?	0	1	2	3	4	5	6

From Izard (1991)

Table 4.2 Ordered logits for emotions in 7 countries from the 2006–2007 European Social Survey

	Happiness	Depression	Anxiety
Bulgaria	−1.8829 (26.66)	0.2715 (3.39)	0.1460 (1.95)
Denmark	0.8112 (12.22)	−0.8543 (9.84)	−2.1782 (25.00)
France	0.2637 (4.28)	−0.1376 (1.88)	−0.3743 (5.48)
Germany	−0.3654 (6.22)	−0.0690 (1.00)	−2.3118 (31.74)
Great Britain	0.0187 (0.31)	−0.2742 (3.78)	−0.8920 (13.19)
Russia	−1.2003 (19.42)	0.3083 (4.36)	0.1851 (2.77)
Spain	0.2956 (4.65)	−0.2762 (3.69)	−1.6832 (22.57)

From Blanchflower (2009)

an emotion and then rate the emotion on dimensions by using the items in Table 4.1.

A variation of the method is the Nobel prize winner Kahneman's "Day Reconstruction Method" (DRM), which is a self-report where persons rate their emotions related to their activities during a day (Kahneman & Krueger, 2006; Kahneman, Krueger, Schkade, Schwartz, & Stone, 2004). The DRM can be administered to large samples and show how life satisfaction and well-being is distributed among different groups in a society (women, men, young, old, rich, poor), or even between inhabitants in different countries. Variations of this method may even lead to "profiling" of the quality of life in different countries by indicating the inhabitants' emotional responses. An example of this is an excerpt from a study of 18 European countries based on the European Social Survey 2006–2007 shown in Table 4.2. The result indicate, e.g. that the Bulgari and the Russians are not very happy but cope reasonably well with sadness (depression) and fear (anxiety), whereas the Danes and the Spaniards are generally happy but also rather anxious.

4.2 The Experience of Physiological Signals

Studies on the experience of signals from the body in emotional experience have aimed as mapping participants' awareness of changes in different parts of the body. The instructions in these studies were that participants should imagine a typical emotional episode and mark on a questionnaire which part of the body that would be affected by the emotion. A notion of the questionnaires may be related to Table 4.3 (see page 27), which shows a simplified version of the results from Wallbott and Scherers (1986, 1988) study with participants from 27 countries.

The results in Table 4.3 show experiences of physiological signals which also were shown as quite similar in participants from different countries (see also Sect. 9.3). A main point of the results is that some emotions, notably happiness, fear and sadness, were associated with several signals in different parts of the body, whereas others, such as disgust and guilt, do not seem to stimulate any specific signals. This does not mean that there is a lack of physiological reactions associated with disgust and guilt or that people are not aware of them, but only that signals from these emotions are not specifically related to the parts of the body in Table 4.3.

It is implied in the results that persons may experience different physiological signals for different emotions. The fact that some changes both are few and may be the same for different emotions shows that there are no specific links from physiological responses to specific emotions such as is implied in the renown JamesLange's theory (see Chap. 11) that emotions are the results of physiological changes (see Sect. 11.2).

Other studies on this issue have shown that there may be large variations between person as regards the number, type and saliency of experienced physiological signals. Some people may experience many and varied signals, while others scarcely note any change at all. There is, moreover, also variation in the extent to which physiological signals are experienced as related to emotions. It is for instance very common to note a lump in the

Table 4.3 Asterixes which mark the experience of physiological signals of 7 emotions

Emotions							
Physiological signals	Happiness	Fear	Anger	Sadness	Disgust	Shame	Guilt
Lump in throat				*			
Breathing		*	*				
Stomach		*		*	*		
Feeling cold		*		*			
Feeling warm	*						
Feeling hot			*			*	
Heartbeat	*	*	*			*	
Muscles tense		*	*				
Muscles relaxed	*						
Perspiring		*				*	
Laughing	*						
Crying				*			
Much talk	*						
Little talk		*		*		*	*

From Wallbott and Scherer (1986)

throat and a fidgety stomach without realizing that this may be a sign that one is sad. Physiological signals of emotions may, on the other hand, also be falsely associated with physiological dysfunction or illness. The sweating and frequent heartbeats which are associated with fear are for instance at times interpreted as indications of heart failure, which tends to arouse additional fear with associated signals (e.g. chest pain) that supports the heart failure interpretation.

4.3 The Intensity Dimension

Researchers have pointed out that emotional experience generally varies in two basic dimensions. The first dimension is valence, which refers to a variation along a positive-negative dimension and is represented by the opposition of positive and negative emotions in Chap. 3.

The second dimension is intensity, and is show in the variation within each emotion in terms of more intense emotional experiences, larger physiological reactions and more marked facial expressions as depicted in Fig. 2.1. Variations in behavior are generally shown in increased quickness and forcefulness, but are also shown in variations in behavior types due to the adaptive challenges in the situation. The variations can be represented by a curve function for the relation between the intensity of the emotion and the effectiveness of its associated behavior. The function is adapted from a description of the relation between motivation and learning by Yerkes and Dodson in 1908, and is depicted in Fig. 4.1 (see page 28).

Figure 4.1 is an illustration that intensity is both a necessary and a sufficient condition of adaptation and that increase in intensity leads to an increase in the efficiency of the behavior until a point where the intensity becomes overwhelming and behavior efficiency deteriorates. A description can be that the lowest level of intensity arouses attention and registration. When the intensity increases, for instance because the attention is focused on an interesting object, one may differentiate more clearly between what is more or less important and evaluate behaviors which might be instigated. A further increase in intensity serves as energy for planning and carrying out a sequence of activities in order to obtain a goal. This is accomplished most efficiently within an optimal zone of intensity indicated in Fig. 4.1. An increase in intensity beyond the optimal zone can lead to an emotional «supercharge» resulting at first in a too focused attention to a part of an event or situation, and a further increase in intensity may lead to tunnel vision, i.e. a focus which is fixated to the extent that there is a loss of awareness of the main task at hand. This is the beginning of a fragmented adaptation, i.e. that the diverse behaviors, perceptions and thoughts that must be coordinated to obtain a goal are no longer related to each other. The highest levels of intensity may even result in a paralysis of coping efforts, as is for instance shown when a person is entering a state of shock under overwhelming threat and stress.

Rescue teams at accidents and fires are familiar with examples of supercharged persons. They have arrived at scenes were intensely scared persons have made disastrous decisions such as jumping from a ship at sea or from the fifth floor in situations which have been scary but not very dangerous. The problem might, for instance have been just a surface fire about to develop which emanated flames that scared persons to the extent that they were not able to connect their sensations to reason and to appropriate behavior. Students' best known examples may be that intense emotion to succeed at examinations have led to a detrimental focus on the description of details and a concurrent loss of overview, or even at times to a blocking ("iron curtain") on the access to the relevant memory.

The optimal zone in Fig. 4.1 (see page 28) represents a high level of intensity which results in a maximum organiza-

Teil I

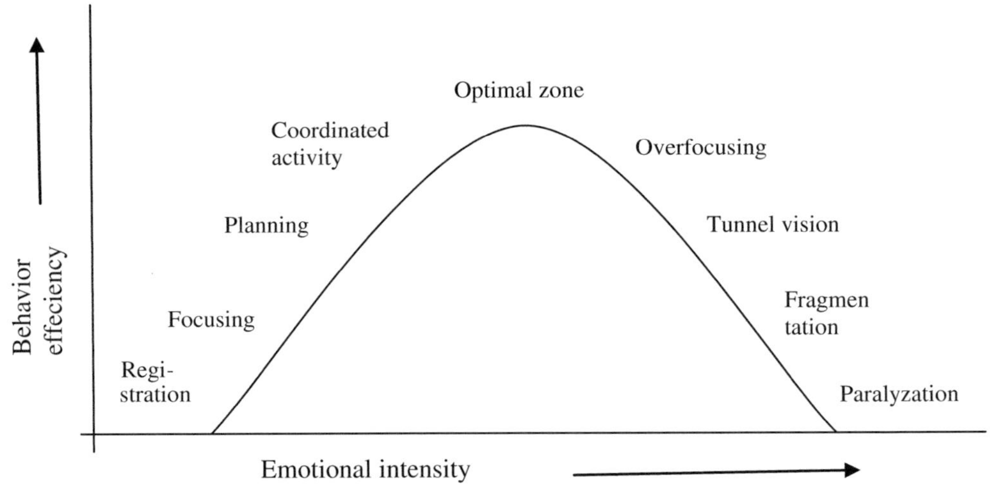

Fig. 4.1 Yerkes-Dodson's law applied to emotions: The relation of behavior efficiency to emotional intensity

tion of task execution. Performance in the optimal zone is the aim of everyone who is dependent on exposed and intensive output, such as stage actors, entertainment artists, athletes and sportswomen and pupils and students at important exams. The obtainment of the optimal zone varies with individual characteristics. Some persons need to build up intensity over some time or to be activated by intensive stimulation, while others may be supercharged almost immediately and need no enhanced stimulation. Optimality also varies with additional factors. One is for instance supercharged more easily when tired than when rested, and more easily in stressful than in quiet situations.

It may be noted that supercharge and supercharged reactions are not limited to negative emotions. The coordination in adaptation is weakened in intensely positive responses. One example is falling in love, which is known to result in tunnel vision and at times to a state similar to psychological paralysis.

4.4 Emotions and the Self. Emotion as Traits and Resonance

The significance of emotions for each person is especially expressed by the fact that emotions are close to, or part of a person's self. The self refers to a person's experience of him-herself and/or her-his "I". There are several views and theories on this issue, a common conception is that emotions are internalized, or internal parts of the self. The self is, for example, assumed to have a built-in emotional component in the form of self-esteem. Self-esteem is defined as a positive or negative emotional attitude that influences a person's acceptance and confidence in herself/himself (see e.g. Larsen & Buss, 2002).

Another example of self-internalized emotions may be that a person's self is formed in close relation to a dominant emotion in terms of a trait. This relates to Spielberger's (1972) distinction of *state anxiety*, which was conceived as a transitory state of responses to a context shown in ordinary adaptation, and *trait anxiety*, which was conceived as a generally high level of anxiety shown (e.g.) in a disposition to respond with anxiety under stress characteristic of persons with anxiety disorders (Endler & Kocovski, 2001). Other emotions which have been generalized as traits are aggression (Bushman, 1995) and shame (Rohleder, Chen, Wolf, & Miller, 2008). The inclusion of emotions as relatively stable components in the self is also suggested in the five basic («Big Five») personality traits of openness, conscientiousness, extroversion, agreeableness, and neuroticism which have turned out in practically all measures of personality (McRrae & Costa, 1990). The emotions which are especially evident in these traits are, respectively, interest, anxiety, happiness, and anxiety and sadness.

An additional internalized emotions is that emotionality is recognized as part of the attitudes which represent a person's basic values and views on the world and herself/himself. All these viewpoints imply that emotions affect how persons represent and present themselves, their ordinary day-to-day adaptation, the goals they set for themselves and their general orientation to others and their being in the world. The significance of this also is that the selective drive inherent in emotions (see Sect. 1.5) may result in biased interpretations of the surroundings and prejudiced behavior if and when the self and its values and views are dominated by the internalized trait for one single emotion, i.e. trait anxiety or trait aggression.

Whereas internalizations are built up during development and functions indirectly, the self is also influenced immediately and directly through emotional resonance, which means that emotions are reflected in a persons' awareness of themselves. A person who, for instance, feels envy may experience this as very disagreeable because he or she may feel unworthy by harboring such a despicable emotion. The resonance of fear and anxiety is known to result in a conception of oneself as little competent, and happiness seems to resonance on the self as positive and valuable. These examples may also show that resonance may increase the pain associated with negative emotions and to increase the pleasure of positive ones.

4.5 Fear of Emotions

Descriptions in this book (see Sects. 1.7, 1.8, and 2.6) have suggested that emotions are aroused without being planned and without conscious control, lead to experiences of unpleasant physiological signals, result in supercharged intensity which results in wrongful and life-threatening decisions and resonate in ways that are directly opposite of the concept we have of ourselves. Thus, emotions may be conceived as unstable and powerful forces which are little accessible and may result in unstable and dangerous conditions. They have in this respect become internal enemies which are feared and which must be opposed with suppression and other form of control.

Internal emotional enemies are often the reason when one feels tense and either avoids or is very reserved and clumsy in relation to other persons. This may be persons that one is actually angry at, or even persons who are conceived as very attractive. The problem is that both "negative" and "positive" persons can provoke intense emotions which results in great uncertainty and lack of control of one's behavior, and the emotions have thus become sources of fear.

Fear of emotions and attempts to control them may be causes both of emotional and somatic health problems (see Chap. 7). And since intense emotions may short-circuit adaptive effort (Sect. 4.3), a slight anxiousness in relation to emotions is probably a general aspect of persons' existence rather than a health problem. This is supported by results from a study where participants responded to a questionnaire about fear of emotions which showed that they feared intense anger and sadness as well as fear and happiness (Williams, Chambless, & Ahrens, 1997). Examples of questions in the questionnaire are shown in Table 4.4.

It can be noted in relation to this and to Sect. 4.3 that results which indicate that variation in emotional intensity and fear of emotions are general aspects of emotions may suggest that sources of emotional problems may be neither the frequency nor the intensity of specific emotions (e.g. sadness or fear). Problems may, rather, be the manner in which persons cope with (see Sect. 7.3) or regulate (see Chap. 8) their emotions.

4.6 Emotion as Community: Emotional Contagion

The three preceding sections were mainly about intrapersonal aspects of emotions, i.e. the persons' relations to his-her emotions. A contrast to this it was shown in the presentation of Dimberg, Thunberg, and Elmehed (2000) study which suggested that emotions can be fundamentally interpersonal by being transferred from one person to another by one person's unconscious registration and imitation of the other's facial expression. This can be conceived as a form of emotional contagion, which has been defined as: "a tendency of automatic imitation and synchronization of facial expressions, sounds/language, body carriage and movement in another person associated with emotions" (Hatfield, Cacioppo, & Rapson, 1994).

The subcortically based imitation in Dimberg et al.'s (op. cit.) study and studies of imitation in newborns supported a viewpoint that emotions are based on inherited neuronal circuits. The results of this research are also supportive of Hoffmans (1990) theory that humans are borne with an empathic relation to each other. These are not new theories. A concept of "emotional imitation" was assumed to be the basis of human community and proposed as explanation of mass behavior by, respectively, Gabriel Tarde in 1890 (Tarde, 2003) and Gustave LeBon in 1895 (LeBon, 1960). The associated concept of emotional contagion has often been offered as an explanation of irrational, fanatical and destructive reactions, for instance of the hostile aggression in participants at political rallies or spectators at football games. But contagion may also be sources of panic in a crowd and the jubilant emotions at rock concerts and religious meetings. The aggressive facial expression of dictators such as Mussolini and Hitler, and the benign expression generally presented by religious leaders may be suggested as real-life examples of Dimberg et al. (2000) study.

Emotional contagion has been documented in several studies. One of the best known was conducted by Bush, Barr, McHugo, and Lanzetta (1989), who used a humor video (Monthy Python type) and had half the participants look at close-up photos of persons who laughed while looking at the video. Contagion was shown when participants with close-up photos showed more happy facial expressions and reported

Table 4.4 Selected questions from a questionnaire about fear of emotions (response is rating on seven point scales of fear of losing control)

Anger:
I am concerned that I will say things I'll regret when I get angry
I am afraid that I will hurt someone if I get really furious
Happiness:
I can get too carried away when I am really happy
I am afraid that I can do something dumb if I get carried away
Sadness:
I am afraid that I can go into a depression that would wipe me out
I am afraid that I might try to hurt myself if I get too depressed
Fear:
I get so rattled when I am nervous that I cannot think clearly
I am afraid that I will babble or talk funny when I am depressed

From Williams et al. (1997)

more merriment than the half of the participants who had looked at the video without close ups. Participants in a similar study observed persons who either described their most happy or most sad memories, and who showed the concomitant facial expressions. Direct observations of participants' facial expressions showed that they were similar to the ones who were observed (Hsee, Hatfield, Carlson, & Chemtob, 1990).

There may be several and diverse consequences of emotional contagion. An example is provided by Coyne's (1976) study, where participating students should get to know a woman by talking with her on the telephone for 20 min. Half of the students talked to a woman who was depressed, and the other half with a woman who had no emotional problems. The results showed that those who had talked to the depressed woman rated themselves as sadder than those who had talked to the woman without problems. Similar results, i.e. that negative emotions may be taken over or infected, have been shown in health workers (nurses and social assistants) whose job is to be empathic and to tune into others, emotions.

An example closer to daily life is salespersons and politicians who try to augment positive emotions in others by their facial expressions and tone of voice to create corresponding emotions related to their products. Another example is variations in the emotional climate at work as a function of salient emotional reactions in one or several colleagues, a third example are variations in the performance of participants on a team influenced by emotions of their coach, team captain, or other central members. There is as yet no agreement between at least six different theoretical position as to how emotional contagion should be explained (Niedenthal, Krauth-Gruber, & Ric, 2006).

4.7 The Need to Talk About Emotions: Social Sharing

It is a widespread assumption that emotions are private and kept outside of the knowledge of other people. Studies conducted by the Belgian professor Bernhard Rime shows that the assumption is false. Emotional experiences seem actually to create a strong need to talk to others about what has happened. Talking about emotions in this way is called "social sharing" by researchers in the area.

An overview after many years of research shows that a person who has experienced an emotion wants to talk to others about this in 80–95% of instances. This is shown by studies whith different methods, in different cultures and geographical areas, and in men as well as in women (Rime, Paez, Kanyangara, & Yzerbyt, 2011). The exception is that the frequency of social sharing is lower for shame and guilt than for other emotions. Reasons for this can be negative resonance of these unpleasant emotions on the self and assumptions that they may show the person in a negative light to others (Finkenauer & Rime, 1998).

A typical Rime-study was a diary study of emotional experiences. Participants described each evening during some weeks their most intense emotional experience during the day, noted their causes and whether the preceding day's most intense experience had been shared with someone (Rime, Mesquita, Philippot, & Boca, 1991). The results showed that sharing in addition to a high base-line frequency was increased by the intensity of the experience. Events which were rated as "very intense" were seen as more important to share with others than experiences rated as "little intense". Results from several studies have, furthermore, shown that the need to share emotions is highest immediately after an event, and that sharing is often repeated by several persons (Rime, 2009). Repeated sharing seems to be regulated by reciprocal acceptance. Persons in general are receptive to emotional sharing even though this leads to some contagion of negative feelings. But there are limits to this receptivity. Persons who have experienced catastrophes or are with life threatening and complicated illnesses may experience that they are avoided after initial contacts because others do not sustain the "burden" of their negative emotions. This may also be examples of the contagious effects shown in Coyne's study in Sec. 4.6.

Rime (2009) has pointed to diverse reasons for the need to share emotions. Firstly, the need may be related to a wish for a repeated experience in order to understand what has happened and one's own and others' responses in the situation. Secondly, sharing may be motivated by a need for understanding, help, support and comfort. Thirdly, sharing serves to create a distance to the experience which may help increase the overview over the event and the control of the concomitant emotions.

Ordinary sharing does not seem to be directly related to health. Rime and co-workers have not, in contrast to Pennebaker's results (see Chap. 6), found that emotional openness in terms of social sharing has had any effect on health. It may be that the generality of sharing means that it is part of an adjustment function rather than a specific therapeutic device for emotional problems. An interpretation has been that emotional sharing is important because emotional experiences are conspicuous and different from the ordinary experiences in persons' daily lives (Rime, Herbette, & Corsini, 2004). They may therefore signal a need for a revision to obtain a shared understanding of the event and its subjective effects in order that the emotional experience can be accepted and interpreted according to a common view of reality. This is supported by results from interviews with persons who have not shared their emotional experiences. They reported that they had been searching for the meaning of the experience over months and years, and that they had made large efforts to understand what had happened in order to establish an order in their experiences (Finkenhauer & Rime, 1998).

4.8 Practical Relevance

The issues in this chapter are all relevant for work with emotional problems, which frequently involve problems in the regulation of emotions such as sadness, fear/anxiety, shame, and guilt. Descriptions of work in this area are provided in books on psychotherapy and in self-help books with information on how to cope with stress and emotional control and to develop self-assertion and self-esteem.

A general development in relation to emotional experiences is to be aware that emotional experiences are just that, i.e. experiences and not a mirror of something outside oneself. This facilitates the insight that one's emotional experience of someone is based both of oneself and the other, and can provide opportunities to discover several other aspects both of you and the other. It also stimulates a differentiation between experience and actual facts which often is necessary to be able to solve misunderstanding and conflicts.

There are many different ways to obtain an optimal level of emotional intensity. This is part of the emotion regulation issue which is discussed in Chap. 8. Emotional regulation is also the main manner of handling fear of emotions. Both issues are targeted in psychotherapy. Fear of fear is always unrealistic, and this may at times be effectively revealed by imagining the worst possible case.

4.9 Summary

Emotional experience is characterized by being directed at something, transforming that which it is directed at and to imply a lack of self-consciousness. This may be a basis for experiences of emotions as revealing some truth.

Emotional experiences comprise signs of physiological changes. Signs are more numerous for some emotions, such as happiness, fear, and sadness, than for others, such as disgust and guilt. There are large individual variations in experiences of such signs, and they may also at times be falsely interpreted as signs of problems in the body rather than as emotional signs.

Emotional experiences vary in intensity and are related to adaptation by a curved function. Increase in intensity is related to increase in adaptive efficiency until an optimal point over which a further increase in intensity leads to a decrease in adaptive efficiency.

Emotions are closely related to and forms part of self and personality. They resonate with the person's self with significance which is associated with the emotion. Negative qualities of emotions such as envy an anger may, accordingly, be established as an internal source of fear because of this reason, i.e. as something that a person do not want to recognize in herself.

Observations and experiments in different groups and interactions have shown that emotions may be contagious. Research has also shown that emotional experiences lead to a need for social sharing, i.e. to get in contact with and communicate with someone.

Reflection Questions

1 Reflect on your adaptation at high intensity levels of interest, happiness, disgust, anger, and fear. Have some of your reactions been related to fear of emotions, for instance fear of how you might feel or respond? Have you experienced being extremely inhibited and/or wanting to avoid or flee when approaching a highly attractive goal? How did you perceive and think, and can you remember any physiological reactions?

2 Emotional contagion is often noticed when one person with a salient emotion arrives in a group and the general emotionality (group climate) changes in the direction of this person's emotion. Has this happened in you study group? In other groups you know? Are contagious responses triggered more easily by specific emotions or by specific persons?

Research/Exercise Examples

1 Studies show that a majority of people want to share their emotional experiences. But why do they want to share? And why should some people avoid sharing? Are there variations in both related to emotion and situation? Design a study to explore these issues.

2 Emotions and the body: How do you feel happiness, anger, fear, and sadness in your body? Make simple A-4 drawings of the front of a body and a head which can be used to register either as a point or an area for a sensation with 1 for "vague", 2 for "clear" and 3 for "intense". Copy the drawings to your study group, use music, pictures or film to stimulate an emotion and do a registration when you can feel the emotion. Also register the intensity of your emotion by a 1–3 rating.

Further Reading

Hatfield, E., Cacioppo, J. T., & Rapson, R. L. (1994). *Emotional contagion*. Paris: Cambridge University Press.

Lambie, J. A., & Marcel, A. J. (2002). Consciousness and the varieties of emotion experience: A theoretical framework. *Psychological Review, 109,* 219–259.

Rime, B. (2009). Emotion elicits the social sharing of emotion: Theory and empirical review. *Emotion Review, 1,* 60–85.

Development of Emotions

5

Emotions were represented in the four first chapters as a standard- or ordinary form which presumably pertains to everybody. But everybody are not students, who were participants in most studies, or other adults. Some are young children and some even infants, and research indicates that at least the youngest ones do not respond emotionally in an ordinary adult form of emotions. A mapping of the development of emotions from their first appearance in newborns is necessary and useful to obtain a full understanding of emotional phenomena, and to obtain some idea of what we bring into this world and how this is changed and established in interaction and communication with other persons.

The focus on development in this chapter means that the text will be concerned with changes in processes and components that results in the coordination of components defined as emotions in Sect. 1.3. The first part in this chapter is among the most difficult ones in this book. The challenge is to understand how a basic biological form is extended to an ordinary form by cognitive processes which must be developed to serve as an extension. The central point is that the developmental problem is resolved by an establishment of a stable anchoring in the child's mind. The stable anchoring is represented by the concept of the object, i.e. by the child's intuitive understanding that the surroundings consists of stable forms or entities which are partly or wholly independent of the child itself. The first indications of this understanding are shown in the ninth to tenth month after birth.

The developmental extension of cognition is shown in this chapter as a change from a diminutive attention in the basic emotions to a very significant cognitive part in the experience of ordinary emotions (see Sects. 1.2, 1.3 and Fig. 1.2). In the course of this time the child becomes aware that the parents' expressions of emotions communicate something, and that he/she can influence the parents in turn. This is represented in this chapter as a development of communication where the child can use emotions as a language, and is shown as the basis of social referencing i.e. the child's learning by observing the parent's emotional responses.

Development of emotions after the first year is described in this chapter as the development of self-conscious emotions from the second to about the fourth year of life. The last part of the chapter comprises a presentation of emotional understanding in the later childhood years.

5.1 The First Year: From Basic to Ordinary Emotions

5.1.1 The First Two–Three Months

It is well documented that facial expressions of emotions are shown in infants practically at birth. A large collection of photographs can, for instance, be found on search for "babies' emotions" and "infants' emotions" on the internet. Photographs with detailed descriptions of expressions are shown in Shaffer (2009). Blind infants show similar expressions as their peers in the first two-three months after birth (Eibl-Eibesfeldt, 1973). Adults have been shown to recognize facial expressions of happiness, interest, and disgust in newborns, expressions of anger, sadness, and fear in the first two-three months after birth and surprise somewhat later. Newborns also express emotions in their voice, for instance by crying and cooing. Fear is shown in behavior as avoidance (turning of the head, avoidance of looking), anger as resistance against being held and interest as orienting responses where the infant stops activities to listen or to fixate her-his glance.

There has been no time and no stimulus for learning the emotional expressions which are shown a short time after birth. It is therefore reasonable to assume that they have been prepared neurologically in the DNA. This is support for a concept of basic emotions and the early warning, subcortically based system which was suggested in Sect. 1.8.

The first emotional reactions are very limited. Researchers have described the early expressions and behaviors as superficial, short-term responses that are more similar to reflexes than to emotional experiences (Saarni, Campos, Camras, & Witherington, 2006). Facial expressions may be little related to the situations, and aroused as often by states in the central nervous systems as by stimuli in the environment. Newborns may, for instance, smile in dangerous situations, and they may smile as often when they sleep as when they are awake. Thus, "inherited" in this context does not mean "adequate" or "complete". There must be large changes in and additions to these first emotional reactions before they become ordinary emotions.

A. Vikan, *A Fast Road to the Study of Emotions*,
DOI 10.1007/978-3-319-52313-2_5

A first and early step in this process is that reactions are systematically related to the environment. Smiles are, for instance, shown as related to voices in the third week after birth, and to visual perception of a person (the mother) in the fourth week (Sroufe, 1996).

Emotional communication. Communication consists of sending and registration of messages. Skills related to both are present at birth. Sending is implied in the emotional expressions as is shown in the attribution of meaning to the newborn's facial expressions ("look how satisfied he is", "she gets angry when…"). Auditory registration is indicated by newborn's weeping when they hear the weeping of other newborns, shows uneasiness and discomfort at high pitched sounds, and reacts differently to neutral, happy, angry, and sad voices (Mastropieri & Turkewitz, 1999). Visual registration is shown by the infants' preference and search of the human face cited in Sect. 2.1, and by the imitation of facial movements which were cited in Sect. 2.6, and is also shown as imitative responses to facial expressions of anger, happiness, and sadness in the first weeks after birth (Meltzoff & Moore, 1983, 1989; Walker-Andrews & Dickson, 1997).

The first communication exchanges consist of the child and the caretaking person (CP, generally the mother or the father) taking turns in signaling interest and attention in relation to each other. Simple examples of this are called "synchronization", and are functioning two months after birth. Signalization is mainly performed by facial expressions. Synchronization consists mainly of facial expressions where each participant, but especially the child, communicates, e.g. what they tolerates and do not tolerate, what they fear and what they like and do not like. Many examples of the emotional content of this communication can be found by searching "mother and baby" and "father and baby" on the internet.

5.1.2 The Experiential Object and Three Types of Emotion

It may seem as a long distance from the basic emotions in Sect. 5.1.1 to ordinary emotions according to the definition of emotions in Sect. 1.3. The changes between the two types are determined by the development of emotional experience. The fleeting reactions in the infant in the first weeks indicate that there is registration of something, but probably no concentrated experience. The contrast is very large as compared to the one-year-old's continuous attention and exploration to the surroundings. Sroufe (1966) and his research group has identified three emotional types or stages between the newborn's and the one-year-old's emotions. A main point of the descriptions is that ordinary emotions refer to the child's realization that the world consists of independent objects, i.e. objects that exist even though the child is not there to perceive them.

The experience of the object.
The newborn's reactions in the first time after birth may not be considered as «proper» experiences because an emotional experience presupposes that it is *about* something (see Sect. 4.1). «Something» in this context denotes an object, and the problem for the newborn is that he/she does not relate to objects. This does not mean that newborns do not see or hear something. They are able to see and hear even before birth, and show recognition of something, for instance their mother's voice, a very short time after birth. But they do not realize that the visual images and sounds refer to solid and independent objects. They have no experience that can tell them that objects such as a cup or a rattle are permanent in time and independent of vision, touch, and the sounds they make. The experienced object is not attributed the qualities of solidity and permanency, and the newborn's perceptions and registrations consequently lack coherence and remain fleeting. The world of the infant is entirely based on the senses, that which is out-of-the eye is also out-of-the-world. A two-three month old infant may for instance lose a rattle or a bottle on the floor and not show any tendency of searching because the object ceases to exist when it is out of sight.

The cognition of objects is dependent on actual experience. Infants lack ability to move around to explore their surroundings, and they have not developed their cognition sufficiently to search for an attractive object (an apple, a rattle) which are taken from them and hidden under a cushion directly in front of them before they are eight-nine months of age. The coherence of experience established by the handling the same objects over time is "stamped" into the child's mind as memories which forms a *subjective basis* for meaning. Thus, one child may laugh to or fear something that elicits no response in others because a stimulus or an event has a specific meaning to this child. This is the background for subjective reactions which, according to Sroufe (1996), are the defining characteristics of ordinary emotions.

Prototypical emotions, precursor emotions and ordinary emotions
A sketch of Sroufe's three types of emotions is shown in Table 5.1 (see page 35). Each type is linked to qualities of the child's experience of objects.

The descriptions in Table 5.1 show differences in the causes of emotions and manner of arousal in emotion in the first year of life. The prototypical reactions (the basic emotions) were described in Sect. 5.1.1. The global, diffuse reactions in precursor emotions refer to responses which are related to stimulation which is «objective», such as a high sudden sound or an intrusive visual stimulus, and triggers responses which are not aimed directly at their cause in children generally. A child who is held tightly may, for instance, flail their arms and legs in anger, but not direct them at the hands which hold her/him. The precursor responses are also often slow and need to be built up. A child may, for instance, not smile at a mask before it has been presented repeatedly, or before he-she has been stimulated by smiling and voice in 30–60 s.

Ordinary emotions are different from precursor emotions mainly by being immediate and aroused by subjective meaning, and by being precise and directed at the cause of the emotion. A one-year-old held tightly will be angry and try to remove the hands that hold her/him. The development of this third type of emotions seem also to be related to rapid

Table 5.1 Key terms for three types of emotions from birth to the last part of the first year

Prototypical emotions. From birth to three months
Facial expressions of six–seven emotions.
Registration of stimulation without object quality ("out of sight, out of mind")
Short term emotional reactions triggered by states in the brain
Precursor emotions. From three- to eight-nine months
Partly built objects which serve expectations and recognition
Global, diffuse reactions to wide classes of stimuli and events
Reactions are triggered by surroundings, but must be built up
Ordinary emotions. From nine months*
Objects are experienced as permanent and independent as shown in searching when they disappear (are hidden)
Reactions are precise and immediate based on subjective meaning (*"Basic emotions" in Sroufe, 1996)

Based on Sroufe (1996)

development of the brain in the infants' first year, especially related to the orbitofrontal area (Schore, 1994) and to the hippocampus in the limbic structure which is central to memory.

5.1.3 Emotional Communication, Analog Emotional Language, and Social Referencing

The development of communication in the first year results in a language and a source of new learning. A beginning can be set to three-month-olds who can recognize a picture of their mother's face among pictures of other faces, and differentiate between emotions in their mother's face and voice. This is the basis for an extension of synchronous routines to verbal dialogues. It is shown initially by infants' smiling and positive sounds in responses to initiatives from CP. 5–6 month old children may include objects, e.g. a ball, and start interactions on their own.

The interaction results in learning that emotional messages may have interesting results. The child is practicing this at about six months of age. Sadness, anger, and happiness can all be expressed in ways that can get CP to satisfy needs, avoid that CP leaves, and/or recruit CP's help with something. This means that emotional expressions have establish relations to references which can be compared to the references of words in ordinary language. The main difference is that the emotional units, i.e. the emotional expressions, are less specific than words, and shows less possibility of message qualification. The limitation is inherent in the analog communication related to facial expressions which was described in Sect. 2.7. Children have become users of an emotional analog language nine months after birth when the development of the object also has served to establish a common focus. A common focus is shown in the child's ability to relate to CP and an object at the same time. The child can, for instance, follow CP's pointing visually and communicate about the same thing. It is part of this development that children are able to control both themselves and others. They know have something can be attained by active and conscious use of emotional signals. Children are, thus, analog users of language long before they are able to use the digital verbal language. This "Emotionese" is mainly based on facial expressions and can be considered as universal (see Chap. 2).

The use of emotions serves as a basis for the development of social referencing. Social referencing is implied in the reference function of emotional communication, and was first shown in a study where 9 month old children were sitting on their mother's lap in a playroom when a new, attention arousing toy (a mechanical ape beating on a drum) was placed on the floor in front of them. The mothers were instructed to show either happiness or fear when the toy was presented, and the children, who remained at the lap the first time, looked at their mother's faces when the toys appeared. The children returned the following day, and the toy was presented again when they were alone in the room. An overview of the study is shown in Table 5.2 (see page 36).

The results showed that children's behavior in relation to the toy was determined by their mothers' emotional expressions. Thus, the reference of the toy was social, i.e. the mothers' emotional expressions, rather than the characteristics of the object itself (color, form). This social referencing is a new and rich source of learning for the child. It means that the child can learn a lot from keeping an eye on others', especially their parents', emotional responses and "read" the meaning of objects, persons, and events without having to experience all this by themselves. This may at times result in responses which are not immediately understood by parents. An example: Mother, who has had some negative experiences in health examinations, meets to health control with her two-year-old-child. She has prepared the child beforehand with positive talk about the occasion. The child reacts in spite of this with attempts to escape and with strong resistance when the health nurse approaches. Mother, who has unconsciously adapted the emotional expression of fear, may be offended and unable to understand the child's behavior.

Table 5.2 Overview of a study of social referencing

General design Two groups of mothers with 9 month old children were instructed to either express happiness or fear in front of an unfamiliar toy
Setup (first day) The mothers sit in a playroom with the children in their laps. An attention arousing mechanical toy (an ape beating on a drum) that the children have never seen are placed on the floor in front
"Happy" mothers were instructed to smile and bend toward the toy "Fearful" mothers wrinkled the eyebrows and stiffened their bodies
Responses The children inspected their mothers' facial expressions
Testing (the following day) Children met with their mothers in the playroom with the mechanical toy and the mother were instructed to leave
Results Children of "happy" mothers crawled toward and examined the toy Children of "fearful" mothers either remained passive at their place or tried to follow their mother

Based on Klinnert (1984)

5.2 The Second Year: Self-conscious Emotions

The development of the object leads to an ability to keep emotional experiences in consciousness over time with sufficient endurance to be recognized as states in the child's internal world. These states, and experiences of being a cause or an "actor" associated with the child's rapidly developing motor skills, may be the center of a "self" with an in-built emotionality which was described in Sect. 4.4. This can mean that children who are often happy may have other qualities built into their self than children whose most frequent experiences have been fear and/or anger.

Researchers agree that the child's experience of a self develops when new emotions appear around the age of 16–17 months, but not about which emotions are the first to appear. Lewis (1993, 2010) held that the first new emotions were embarrassment, envy, empathy and jealousy, while others have pointed to shame (Schore, 1994; Sroufe, 1996) . The differences probably relate to differences in interpretations of the child's behavior, but envy and jealousy are actually advanced states that presuppose cognitive developments which are not present until the third- or fourth year of life. All these emotions, with the exception of empathy (which is not an emotion) are called "self-conscious" emotions because their reference is a self, and because they cannot be developed without a self. They are also called «social» because they are developed long after birth, do not show universal facial expressions and seem to be developed as a result of the child's social interaction (see Sect. 1.9). The core of self-conscious emotions is the discovery that one is "somebody" who is being perceived by another person.

Emotional communication is developed in the second year of life by the use of analog language to start and maintain play with peers. The interaction is dominated by reciprocal imitation until about 18 months of age. Children at this age start reversing roles by, for instance, one running in front of the other, stopping and turning and having the other run in front. It is about this age that the first references to emotions are shown in children's language in terms such as "happy", "sad", "angry", "afraid", "likes" and "dislikes" (Bretherton, McNew, & Beeghly-Smith, 1981).

5.3 Development in the Third to Fourth Year

The development most related to emotions in the third year of life is children's ability to conceive of themselves as responsible for their behavior and its consequences. This is the background for pride and guilt, which were called "self-evaluating emotions" by Lewis (2010). Examples of pride are children between 2½ and three years of age who look to others and are evidently proud when they have completed a puzzle (Stipek, 1995). Examples of guilt are three-year-olds' uneasy reactions and tendencies of confess when they have been doing something they shouldn't. Guilt refers to an internalized standard for "good" and "bad" and for "correct" and "faulty".

There is a lack of direct studies of the first examples of other emotions, such as envy and jealousy. A general assumption is that all emotion types are developed when the child is about four years old.

5.4 Further Development

The changes after the age of four years concern the expression, intensity, and frequency of different emotions. The expression is changed as a function of self-observation, self-control, and learning of emotional rules (see Sect. 8.2). Adolescence, which is known for its intense emotions and frequent and varied emotional arousal, is an example of changes in intensity. Other age periods, such as the time period for establishing a partnership, a family, becoming a parent, seeing the children leaving home and having grandchildren, imply changes in the intensity and the frequency of different emotions, such as happiness, anger, sadness, and fear. Emotions will also be enriched by new experiences and new memories in all phases of life. The happiness of a 14-year-old is different from the happiness of a person of 44 years of age. This means that emotions also may be conceived as a process in constant change and development throughout the life span.

5.5 Understanding Emotions

Understanding of emotions has become a relevant issue because emotions have shown that this is important both for health and for behavior in organizations. Development of understanding is generally discussed under headlines "empathy" and "component in understanding".

The development of empathy. Empathy is defined as a vicarious emotional response, and refer to a person's understanding of another person's emotions by taking part in them (Vikan, 2006). It was mentioned in Sect. 4.4. that newborns respond with crying to each other's weeping. Hoffman (1990) conceived this as an example of a primary empathic relation. In the two first stages in his four stage model of the development of empathy Hoffman proposed that children empathize with other persons' emotions without differentiating between herself/himself and the other. Children in the first stage may, for instance, seek support to alleviate their own emotion after having been empathically aroused (infected) by another, and children in the second stage who is aroused by another's emotion may offer some of their own things (or their mother) as support. It is in a third stage about three years after birth that children may show a genuine understanding of another's emotions by realizing that other persons may experience situations different from themselves, be aroused by a different emotion and need a support which is specific to the other. A fourth stage begins according to Hoffman (1990) when the child is 10–12 years and comprises an ability to understand how others' emotions are related to their situation in life.

Components in the understanding of emotions. Maps of children's understanding of emotions has been based on observations of behavior, experiments, tests and interviews related to visual illustrations (films, pictures). Observations have shown practical understanding of emotions in two- and three-year-olds in terms of ability to tease and to comfort others' emotions (Dunn, 1994). As "understanding" is a very wide concept, development has been described, alternatively, in terms of eight skills of emotional competence (Saarni et al., 2006) or nine components (Pons, Harris, & DeRosnay, 2004).

Saarni et al.'s (2006) skills are described as frames of emotional development where emotional insight is related to personal and social adjustment from the first years of life until adolescence and beyond. Skill 1, "Awareness of one's own emotional state", is, for instance, shown to be central for setting goals, formulate plans and resolving relationship conflicts. The skill is held to appear for the first time in 2 and 3 year olds talk about how they feel, and be elaborated by insights into causes and consequences of their emotion in the fourth year fifth year of life. A recurring theme in Saarni et al.'s (2006) discussions is reference to studies whose results have shown that children with emotional and social problems show delays and/or biases in their emotional understanding.

Pons et al.'s (2004) components are related directly and specifically to emotional understanding and to actual studies, and are therefore shown in an overview in Table 5.3 (see page 38). Age indications are only gross indications to when a component has been shown to appear or to be developed in a majority of children.

The descriptions in Table 5.3 indicate that understanding starts from about the age of three. There are, however, also results from studies which show examples of understanding in addition to the practical insight noted in the introduction to this section. Children between two and three years of age have, for instance, been shown to know which words refer to different emotions in descriptions of happiness, anger, sadness, and fear (Banerjee, 1997), and to talk spontaneously about their own and others' emotional states (Saarni et al., 2006). There are also studies which show that children in this age may differentiate between pleasant and unpleasant emotions. Understanding of envy and jealousy depends on complex cognition regarding person's relationships to each other and is not generally present before the age of seven (Harris, 1989).

It may be commented on the components in Table 5.3 that the understanding of others' needs (component 3) is basic because it comprise the insight that the same stimulus or situation may arouse different emotions and reactions, such as an insight that Martha may like fish and wants more while Peter hates is and refuses to eat. This insight is also implied in component 4. Component 5 is an example of genuine psychological understanding by representing an insight that something is processed in another person's consciousness. Note that the first development of this is set to a period of three years.

Component 6 will be described further in Chap. 8. Component 8 is based on Harter's (1983) series of studies on children's understanding of the experience of simultaneous emotions. Results from these studies have suggested that children up to five years of age are convinced that it is only possible to experience one emotion in relation to someone or something at a time. Six- and seven-year-olds think that it is possible to harbor different types of emotions for the same object, but only sequentially. It is only from about the age of eight that children realize that they may feel two different emotions for the same object or person at the same time.

5.6 Practical Relevance

The first practical indication in this chapter is associated with the infant's early imitation, which may also be a form for early learning. The fact that imitation is a child's primary manner of learning suggests that this is an effective process for

Table 5.3 Overview of nine components in children's understanding (Un) of emotions

1. *Recognition at about* 3–4 *years.* Skill in recognize basic emotions such as happiness, anger, fear, and sadness from pictures of faces
2. *Un of causes (from about* 3 to 4 *years).* Un that losing a toy or receiving a gift may result in, respectively, guilt and happiness. Comprises Un that different emotions lead to different behaviors
3. *Un of needs and wishes (from* 3–5 *years).* Beginning of Un that persons have emotions that are independent of their needs
4. *Un of belief at about* 3–5 *years.* A beginning realization that behavior is related to a person's belief about something
5. *Un of reminders (between 3 and 6 years).* Un that emotions are related to memories in a way that emotions can be aroused by reminders of what has happened
6. *Regulation of emotions (from about 4–6 years).* Proposal of emotion regulation strategies, i.e. « playing with someone » in order to stop being sad
7. *Hiding of emotions (from about 4–6 years).* Beginning realization that the real emotions can be hidden by misleading expressions, such as smiling when one is actually disappointed
8. *Un that different emotions can be experienced at the same time (from about 8 year).* Un that different emotions can be simultaneous in relation to the same person
9. *Morality (from about 8 years).* Eight-year-old children can begin Un that emotions are related to moral values. i.e. that morally negative behavior leads to negative- and morally positive emotions to positive behaviors

Based on Pons et al. (2004)

establishing and reinforcing social skills. It is therefore a useful practical suggestion to be conscious of imitation both for one's own adaption and as an advice to other persons about how they might learn emotional and social skills. It may also be useful to be conscious of children's tendency to imitate and be a good model for one's own children. This is especially important in relation to the use of facial expressions, which have a key role in communication. The relevance of this is that the maintenance of trustful relationships depends on the clarity of communication between the partners.

It may also be useful to be aware that social referencing is not a source only of children's learning, but a general influence in interpersonal behavior. We inform ourselves as much by other person's emotional expressions as by what they say. And we should be aware that we are all sources of referential communication, i.e. that our emotions are noted and reacted to by others. An advice may be that if you do not understand others' responses to yourself you should reflect on what emotions you may communicate to others.

There are several books on how children are best stimulated to develop empathy and understanding of emotions. The main point in this literature is how children's emotions are met by their parents. An example may be characteristics which have been noted as examples of parents who are good instructors of children's emotions: They are attentive to their children's emotions, conceive of emotions as possibilities of closeness and advice, listen empathically, confirm the children's emotions, help them articulate emotions in words, set limitations on the expression of the emotions and help their children to find strategies to cope with problems (Gottman & DeClaire, 1997).

5.7 Summary

Emotional expressions are present at birth and may be an indication that emotions are basic and inherited forms. Expressions and other reactions are, however, brief, superficial, not related to context and are often aroused by states in the brain in the first two months after birth. The basis of emotional communication is also present at birth as shown in responses to others voices and in imitation of facial movements. Simple exchanges called synchronous routines are established about two months after birth.

An experience of the object is developed as a result of interaction and learning in the first 8–9 months of life. This is the foundation of ordinary emotions, which according to Sroufe (1996) is a third type of emotions in the child's first year of life. Ordinary emotions are preceded by basic proto-emotions in the first two-three months- and precursor emotions between the ages three- and eight months.

The experience of the object and development of communication results in the attribution of meaning to emotional expressions. This leads in turn to an analog language where emotional expressions serve as signs parallel to the function of words in ordinary, verbal languages. Social signals, such as facial expressions, may then be part of a social reference which opens a new source for children's learning.

Self-conscious emotions, such as shame, guilt, and pride, are developed from about 1½ to 3 years after birth. These emotions are often referred to as "social" rather than "basic" emotions because they are developed long after birth and are not shown in universal facial expressions.

Understanding of emotions is developed in several stages and component from the pre-school years. The most basic components, such as the insight that different persons may have different emotions in the same situation, is beginning to be shown in the age phase from 4 to 6 years.

Reflection Questions

1. Be an imaginary small child: Look at people around you and notice their faces, voices and bodies when they engage in some task and/or interact with each other. How would you make sense of that when you do not know emotions?
2. Be an imaginary child of thee-four years of age whose fear, sadness, or anger has become unbearably intense. How would your experience that, what would you need, and how would you react?

Research/Exercise Examples

1. Do some people-watching of children's emotional responses in a kindergarten. Try to characterize the general emotionality of their behavior (are they more or less emotional in their behavior than you and your friends?), their emotional expressions and their emotional control. Control for differences related to gender
2. What are the causes of emotions in children? Do a test of this with a sample of kindergarten and a sample of third grade children, and ask for causes of two basic (e.g. happiness and fear) and two social (e.g. pride and envy) emotions. Be aware that you should test for recognition (ask directly if they are afraid, angry, or sad when…) as well as recall (a simple question about what makes you afraid, angry, etc.)

Further Reading

Lewis, C., & Mitchell, P. (Eds.). (1994). *Children's early understanding of mind*. Hillsdale, N.J: Lawrence Erlbaum.

Saarni, C., Campos, J. J., Camras, L. A., & Witherington, D. (2006). Emotional development: Action, communication, and understanding. In N. Eisenberg, W. Damon, & R. Lerner (Eds.), *Handbook of Child Psychology* (6th ed., Vol. 3, pp. 226–300). New York: Wiley.

Sroufe, L. A. (1996). *Emotional development*. Cambridge: University of Cambridge.

Emotion and Cognition

6

Emotions have been considered as threats to reason from Plato and Aristotle to modern thinking. In this chapter comprises modern studies and discussions on how «reason», in terms of cognition, is influenced by emotion. The first part of the chapter concerns the opposite influence, i.e. how cognition leads to emotions. The second part of the chapter deals with studies and discussions on the "classical" assumption, i.e. that emotions influence cognition in terms of memory, attention, perception, evaluation, and reasoning. A recent approach of studying cognition of emotional processes in terms of emotional intelligence has mainly been developed in relation to applied questions in the workplace, and is referred in Chap. 10.

6.1 Emotions as Result of Cognition: Appraisal Theory

It may seem self-evident, as was referred to in Sect. 1.6, that something must be perceived to be felt, which means that anger, happiness and fear depend on the perception and interpretation of an event. The discussion in Chap. 1 showed that emotion may have other causes than cognition. But cognition is undoubtedly a very important, and probably the most frequent, cause of emotions. Insights into emotions can, therefore, be gained by studies on how they are caused by cognition. This has been the target of researchers who have asked what cognition actually does i.e. how something is appraised as a basis of emotions. An example is Lazarus and Alfert's (1964) pioneering study.

6.1.1 Lazarus and Alfert's Study

The set up for the study was that participants (students) were shown a short anthropological film from the circumcision of adolescent boys in an African tribe. The facial expressions of the adolescents were blurred, but indicated pain or fear. The participants assisted the film in two groups at two different times, and received information about the content of the film beforehand. Participants' emotions were tested by physiological measurement (GSR), and by a questionnaire about their experiences during and after the film.

The information about the film was different for the participant groups. The first group was told that they would see a film of a painful circumcision ritual which the adolescents' had feared in several months. The purpose of the circumcision was told be an opportunity for the adolescents to show that they could behave like men and endure pain. There was, therefore, no attempt to support the boys during the ritual. The second group of participants was told that the film would show a ritual the boys had been looking forward to a long time because it would give them the status of adults. The ritual might seem dramatic, but the boys were offered support and help by experienced elders in the tribe. An overview over the study is shown in Table 6.1 (see page 42).

The results showed that the same stimulus (the film) led to very different emotional responses in the two groups. The participants in the first group showed clear indications of arousal on the physiological measures and reported that they had experienced emotions such as fear or anger during and after the film. The participants in the second group showed only unclear indications of arousal, and reported the experience of positive emotions such as happiness or interest during and after the film. The only difference between the two groups was the difference in information which was provided before the film was shown. Lazarus and Alfert concluded that this information led to differences in participants' appraisal of the film's content, and that the appraisal served as the cause of participants' emotional responses. Appraisal was defined as: "*Evaluation of the significance of something in relation to a person's adaptation in the environment*".

Lazarus and Alferts study and interpretations stimulated a variation in theories and studies classified as appraisal theory. Lazarus and co-workers differentiated between a *primary appraisal*, which consists of an immediate and rough classification of a stimulus or event as «good» or «bad», and a *secondary appraisal* consisting of an evaluation in terms of three components: (a) Attribution of cause and responsibility for the stimulus or event, (b) the possibilities of coping in the new situation, and (c) expectations about further events. This suggests a causal sequence shown in Fig. 6.1 (see page 42).

A. Vikan, *A Fast Road to the Study of Emotions*,
DOI 10.1007/978-3-319-52313-2_6

Table 6.1 Overview of Lazarus and Alfert's (1964) study

Set up	
Two groups of participants received different information about the content of a film which showed a circumcision ritual	
Group 1	Group 2
Instruction	
The film shows a dangerous and painful ritual The boys received no support during the ritual	The film shows a ritual for passage to adult status The boys had support and help from experienced adults
Results	
Participants reacted with negative emotions High physiological arousal	Participants reacted with positive emotions Little physiological arousal

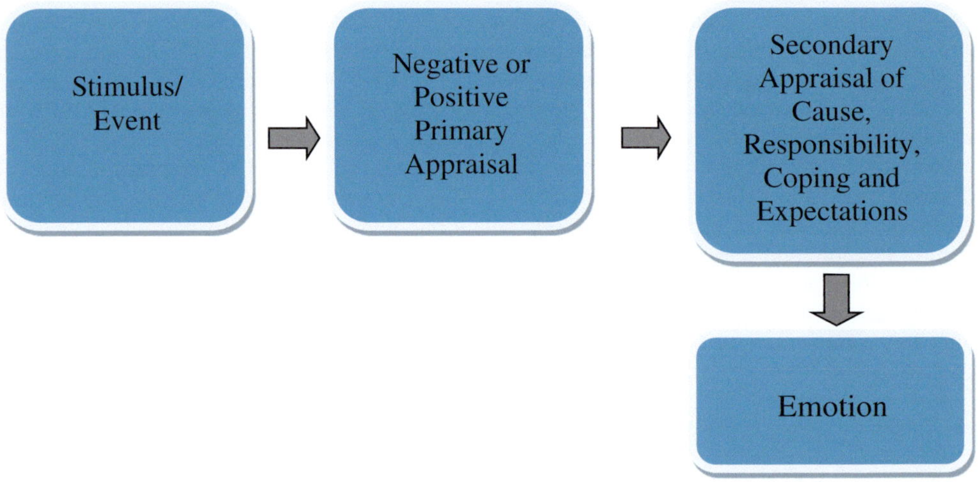

Fig. 6.1 Appraisal in the causal sequence of emotion

An example of the model may be that you are taking a walk in the forest and perceives an animal between the trees. This may lead to a primary appraisal that the animal is dangerous. Your secondary appraisal may be that the animal (*the cause*) is moving freely and is therefore responsible, that *coping* only can consist of leaving the situation and that the *expectation* is that you might be attacked. The resulting emotion is fear. You might, on the other hand, make a secondary appraisal that you will have no difficulty in managing this animal and that it will flee from you. The resulting emotion in this case is anger or contempt.

6.1.2 Dimensions of Appraisal

Appraisal theory is based on the idea that you can predict persons' emotions if you know their appraisals. This should lead to overviews on links between concrete situations and their appraisal, which can be further related to behavior associated with specific emotions. This may seem complicated, but the links are parallel to those that are used in ordinary life. Anne, who is interested in Peter, knows for instance how to manage Peters' appraisals in ways that results in interesting emotions and behaviors. She invites him to her house for dinner, selects a good wine, dims the lights and connects to pleasant music. She assumes that this will result in appraisals in Peter which is associated with positive emotion, and that the emotion will be a selective driver of behaviors in Peter which are positive and pleasurable for Anne.

Attempts to establish overviews have been made by using questionnaires about the causes and extent of different emotions to establish the dimensions of appraisal. An example is a study where participants rated the extent of emotional experiences on 11-point rating scales related to a variation in 15 dimensions (Ellsworth & Smith, 1988; Smith & Ellsworth, 1985). The experiences were tested by questions (rating items), and were rated from "not at all" to "extremely much". Examples of items for rating dimensions of security (a) and control (b):

(a) "To what degree did you feel that you understood the situation around you when you were (happy, angry, afraid, etc.)?"
(b) "To what degree did you feel that factors outside the situation were domineering when you were (happy, angry, afraid, etc.)?"

Statistical analyses of ratings in different studies have yielded somewhat different results. Four dimensions have consistently emerged as decisive for the type of emotion which is experienced in a situation. This is *valence* (the degree of positivity/negativity), *security* (the degree of knowledge), *effort* (the degree of effort needed to reach a goal), and *responsibility* (the degree of responsibility or causation for an event).

It may seem far-fetched to assume that there is no emotion before stimuli or events are appraised in relation at least four dimensions. Researchers have argued that this is no problem because checks on the dimensions are extremely rapid and automatic, and appraisals are only superficially related to typical aspects of a situation after long experience in similar conditions. Another argument is that emotion is not a direct result of appraisals but is part of an appraisal process where information is checked against a number of dimensions (Scherer, 1993, 2001). Yet another argument is a proposal that appraisal can be differentiated into a «basic» type consisting of simple and inherited mechanisms, and a more extensive «cognitive» type related to several dimensions (Frijda, 1993, 2007).

6.2 Cognition as Result of Emotion

The content of Plato, Aristotle and many others' distrust of emotions was that emotions were conceived as negative influences on cognition. There may be some support in this from our daily life. Most of us have probably experienced that we do not function well socially, in interview situations or at different tests when we are very nervous. We may on the other hand also have experiences that there has been little learning and little cognition without some emotional energy, as is evident in the Yerkes-Dodson function in Fig. 4.1. These diverse observations show that there is a need for systematic research before there can be any conclusion about the effects of emotion on cognition.

A first problem on doing research in this area is to select a measure for cognition. Measures may be the ability to remember, evaluate, perceive or reason logically. A second problem is to select which emotions should be tested. Plato and Aristotles' distrust was related to emotions generally, but it may be extremely difficult to check on this by testing all emotions, for example all ten emotions on the list in Table 1.3.

A third problem is how to arouse emotions when participants' are engaged in a cognitive task. A simple and inventive way may be to test persons who are known to have a specific emotion. An example is a study by Forgas and Moylan (1987), who interviewed persons immediately after they had either seen a comical or tragic film, and who consequently were either, respectively, happy or sad (see Sect. 6.2.3). The most frequently used method has been to induce participants into emotional experienced by hypnosis, film/video, music or stories (see Coan & Allen, 2007).

6.2.1 Effect of Emotions on Memory

Congruence

Memory has been one of the most frequently used indicators of cognition in studies on emotion and cognition. The pioneering study was reported by Bower (1981), who employed hypnosis to induce happiness or sadness in participants. One of the tasks was to recall pleasant and unpleasant episodes from participants' childhood when participants were hypnotically induced to be happy or sad. Another consisted of learning a list of words in the morning while hypnotically induced by an emotion, and to recall the list in the afternoon while hypnotically induced to the same or another emotion as the one which was induced during the learning of the list.

Results from Bower's study are shown in Fig. 6.2 (see page 44). The graph to the left shows that participants recalled more unpleasant episodes from their childhood when they were induced as sad than happy, and more pleasant when they were induced as happy than sad. The graph also shows that the differences in memory for unpleasant and pleasant events was larger when participants were happy than when they were sad.

The graph to the right in Fig. 6.2 shows that the memory was best when the emotion under learning the list was the same as the emotion under recall. Those who were happy while learning the list recalled better when they were happy than those who recalled the list when they were sad. And learning and recall when sad resulted in better recall than learning when sad and recalling when happy. The results also suggest that the recall will be better in a person who was either happy or sad during learning than when there was no specific emotion. The morals from the study are that one should be with same emotion when recalling something as one was during learning.

The concordance between emotions at learning and recall was interpreted as the most efficient condition for memory functioning and called "congruence" and "the congruence hypothesis" by Bower (1981). Congruence can imply that cognition may serve to reinforce and enlarge an emotion. Our happiness may, for instance, be reinforced and enlarged because it provokes the memory of pleasant memories. This is a positive effect, but congruence may be a problem when it serves to reinforce and enlarge negative emotions such as sadness, anger, and fear. The effect may, for instance, lead to the negative evaluations of the past, the future, and oneself which is a characteristic of depressed persons (Clark & Beck, 1999). Congruence may also be part of anxiety disordered patient's tendency of exaggerate the dangers in the surroundings (Clark, 1999).

The congruence hypothesis has been supported by the results from many subsequent studies, but it is not clear if it is also effective for emotions such as interest, disgust, shame, and guilt. It is also not clear whether the effect vary with the type of the emotion and/or with the type of data which is recalled (Miranda & Kihlstrom, 2005; Niedenthal, Krauth-Gruber, & Ric, 2006).

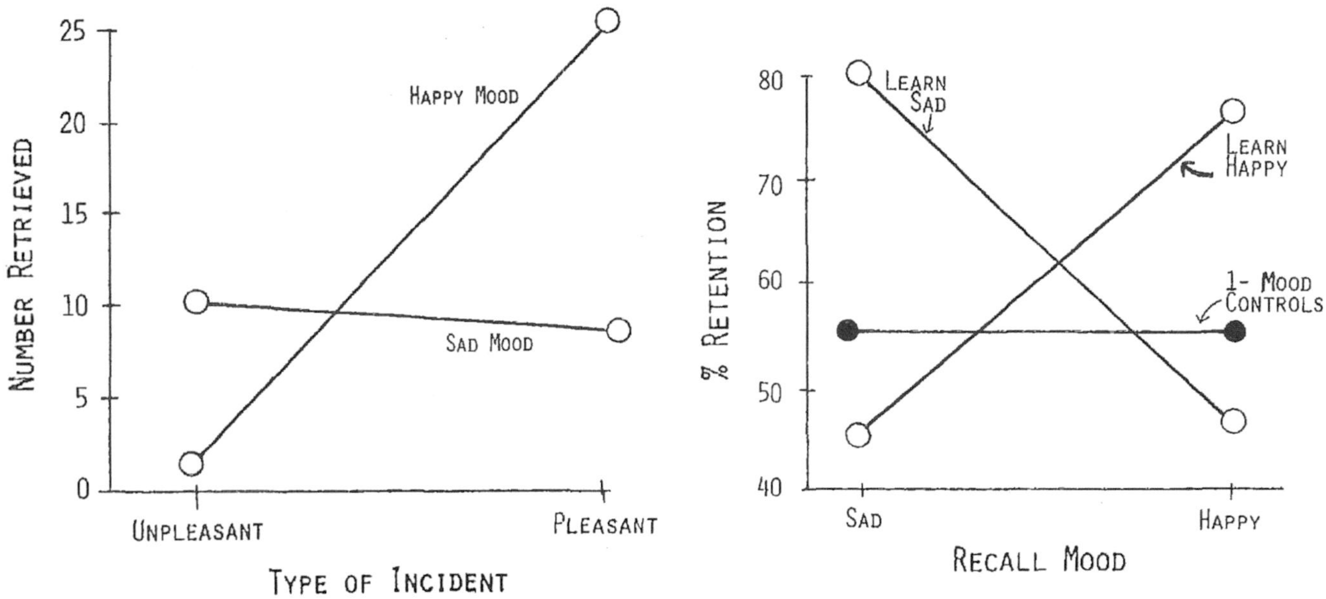

Fig. 6.2 Graphs of results which show emotion-related recall of childhood events (*left*) and retention of word list (to the *right*) (from Bower, 1981)

Intensity of the Experience
Congruence shows that memory is influenced by qualitative variations (emotion types). Memory may also be influenced by quantitative variations i.e. variations in emotional intensity. Quantitative variations are difficult to induce. Studies have, therefore, been related to the memory of events which arouse intense emotions. Results from these studies have suggested that high intensity experiences results in very clear and inclusive recall. An example may be Yuille and Cutshall's (1986) interview of 13 persons two days- and again two–three months after they were witnesses to murder. The witness responses showed 93% accuracy of recall at the first-, and 88% recall at the second interview.

Similar high percentages of recall have been shown for studies of «flashbulb» memory. This is memory for sudden, salient, and negative common experiences, such as the murders of president Kennedy and Martin Luther King and the 9.11 attack in New York. It seems that events which arouse intense emotions by being experienced as painful and threatening may be «burnt into» consciousness and memory. Memories may then be a problem as part of a traumatic stress disorder by appearing suddenly outside of a person's control with images («flashbacks») which may restart the original and intense emotions.

Close examination has shown that memory for intense experiences are not necessarily very clear for all parts of the experience. Analyzes on this point has been related to a differentiation between central and peripheral information. Central information pertains to that part of a stimulus or event which is directly related to an emotion and peripheral information pertains to all other information in a situation. Examples can be related to two photographs which have been employed in studies in this area and which are shown in Fig. 6.3 (see page 45). The top photo shows an emotional event where a badly harmed, blood-stained child provides the central information. The peripheral information in the picture is part of the front window with windscreen wiper and parts of a wheel and a headlight. The bottom picture is a control stimulus which is not selected for emotionally arousing qualities.

Results from the study with the photographs in Fig. 6.3 showed that participants remembered much more details from the top- than from the bottom photograph, and that the remembered details were mainly from the central information. The results also showed that information from the bottom photograph was in fact better remembered than the peripheral information in the upper one. It may, thus, seem that emotions direct attention as a beam of light in intense situations. The information inside the beam is remembered while information outside is forgotten. The set up for the study may be a parallel to situations which arouse intense negative emotions (fear or anger) in witnesses. This may lead to "tunnel vision" where witnesses only note the central information. It is important to be aware that witnesses to events which arouse intense emotions may show reliable recall only for central parts of the event. Knowledge of how memory is influenced by emotions is, therefore, part of a witness psychology which relevant in the daily proceedings in court in many countries.

The relation between intensity and memory may be straightforward in simple, transparent situations. Results from studies have shown that the relation is complex in situations where there are room for different interpretations and meaning. The memory for sexual abuse may, for instance, be very sketchy both in victim and perpetrator because this is a subject which is associated with shame. Results from studies with a focus on happiness suggest that memory for positive events are less related to central information and result in less recall than memory for negative events (Levine & Pizarro, 2006; Peace & Porter, 2004).

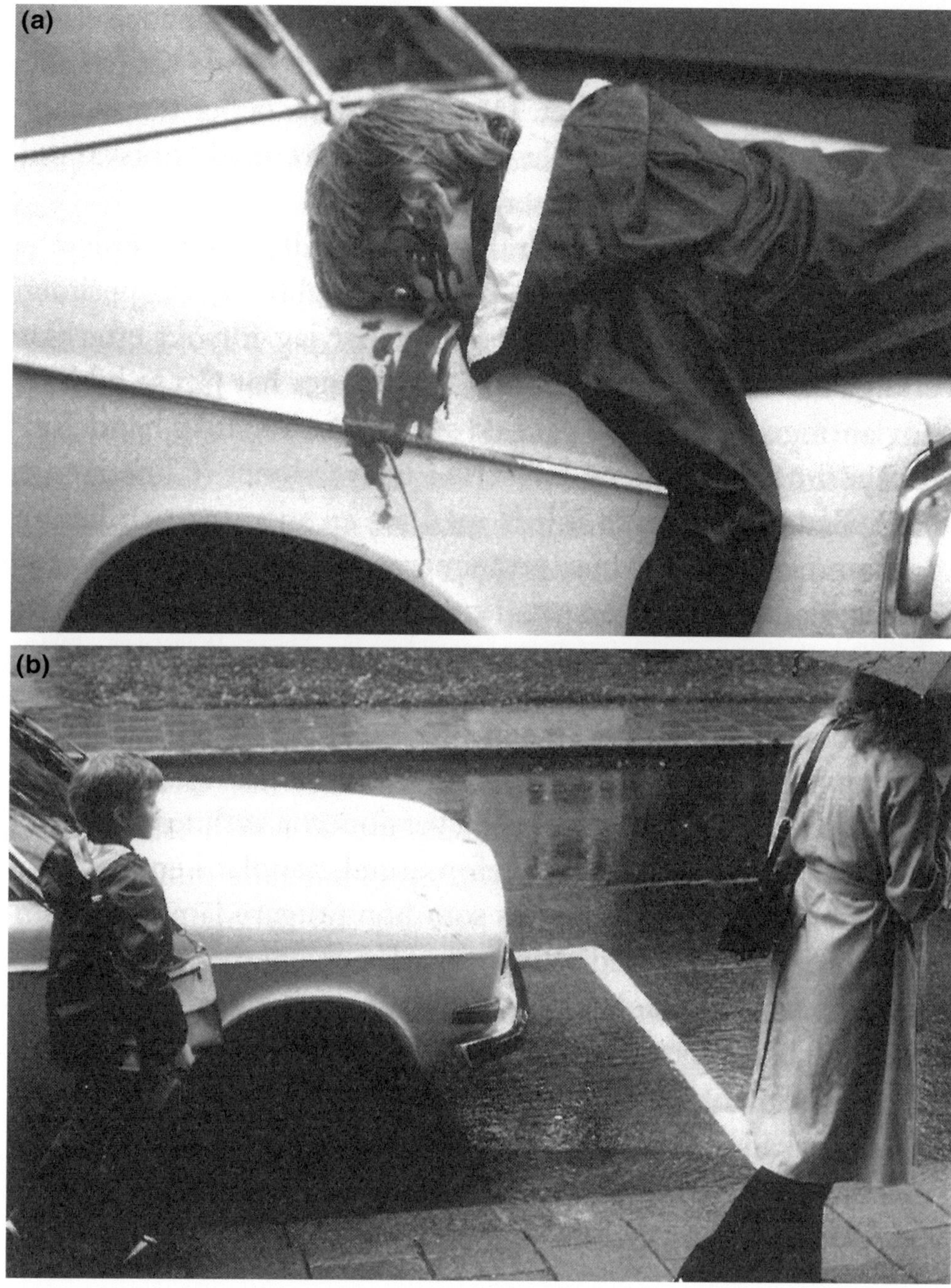

Fig. 6.3 Photo used in testing recall of central and peripheral information (*top* **a**) and a non-arousing control-photo (*bottom* **b**) (from Christianson, 1994)

6.2.2 Effect of Emotions on Other Cognitive Processes

Attention and Perception

Emotion's selective drive implies that emotions functions selectively for attention and perception. Fear leads to a search for and an attention to stimuli which may seem threatening or be part of some danger, surprise directs the attention towards something which was not expected, anger directs attention to opponents, etc. Support for this is provided by results from studies which have shown that emotionally arousing stimuli always receives more attention than neutral ones, and that attention, consequently, seems to function according to a congruence principle (Yiend, 2010). Modern studies are often conducted by use of the «morphing» method, which is a data program where facial expressions for positive and negative emotions are arranged on a dimension. One may, for example, start with a neutral face, click one time and see the same face a little changed but still neutral, click one more time and see the same face still as neutral but at the same time slightly sad, etc. Examples are found by searching "morphing faces" on the Internet. The method serves to measure differences in recognition of emotional expressions. One person may, for instance, only need three clicks from neutral to identify sadness, whereas another may need five or six. A further example may be that results from a study by Niedenthal, Halberstadt, Margolin, and Innes-Ker (2000) showed that happy and sad persons perceived, respectively, more happy and sad pictures than persons without a specific emotion.

Evaluation and Reasoning

Congruence has been repeatedly shown in studies on evaluation and reasoning. An example is Forgas and Moylan's (1987) study, which was mentioned in Sect. 6.2, and which showed that persons who had assisted a comedy were happy and yielded positive evaluations of politicians, measures against criminality, and themselves. Persons who had assisted a dramatic film, on the other hand, were a little sad and yielded slightly negative evaluation of politicians, measures against criminality and themselves. Other examples are that angry persons have been shown to assume higher possibility for provoking situations than sad persons, and that fear increases- and anger decreases evaluations of risk to die from some illness.

Results from studies on how persons reach decisions and interpret unclear situations have also conformed to congruence. Persons who are anxious imagine more dangerous possibilities and select more low-risk alternatives than non-anxious persons. Positive emotions have, furthermore, shown to be related to high risk- and sadness to low risk alternatives (Blanchette & Richards, 2010).

A question which may arise from studies such as these is if they really show that congruent alternatives are actually caused by the emotions. An alternative interpretation of the results is that they refer to the cognitive component of the emotions, and that evaluations of risk and unclear situations are not causes of emotions but a part of the emotional arousal. The results may in these cases only be interpreted as confirmations of the selective drive function of emotions (see Sect. 1.5).

What is needed for a clearer view in this instance is a better differentiation of emotion and cognition in the set-up of studies. This can be achieved with structured descriptions of cognitive functions and/or tested in relation to structured cognitive tasks. This has been part of the set up in tests of the effects of positive (happiness) and negative (sadness) emotions, and has been conducted by Isen and co-workers' research on positive emotions (Isen, 2004; Isen, Daubman, & Nowicki, 1987). The results from this research were that happiness was related to flexible, creative, far-reaching, and original modes of thinking, as well as by a top-down, deductive reasoning. Results from other studies have indicated that happiness also can lead to reasoning with a low degree of self-criticism, simplified and stereotypic viewpoints and heuristic rules.

Table 6.2 Reasoning when happy and sad

Happy	Sad
Far reaching and original	Conservative and systematic
Flexible and creative	Analytical and thorough
Top down deductive	Bottom up inductive
Simplified and superficial	Depressive and realistic
Use of stereotypes	Empiricism

Sadness has, by comparison, been related to a conservative, systematic reasoning which is analytic, empirical and bottom-up inductive. This sad attitude may be the preferred one when it is necessary to be analytic and thorough and avoid misleading and attention-arousing blind alleys. This reasoning has also been called "depressive realism", and constitutes a contrast to the somewhat superficial reasoning which is stimulated by positive emotions. An overview of «happy» and «sad» thinking is provided by Table 6.2.

There is little knowledge and very few studies on reasoning related to other emotions. It has been proposed that anger and disgust may lead to a top down thinking similar to the one in happiness because these emotions, like happiness, are high confidence emotions. Fear has been proposed to have parallel effects on reasoning to that of sadness because it is a low confidence emotion with a need to examine the surroundings in an analytical and thorough way.

Judgment, especially as in terms of economic decision-taking and estimation of risk, has been the subject of voluminous research. The main target has been the effect of cognitive biases (Kahneman, 2011) , but it has been recognized that emotions may serve as information in judgments generally (Loewenstein, Weber, Hsee, & Welch, 2001; Schwartz, 2001) Systematic research has been related to the pleasant-unpleasant dimension with results corresponding to those which are summarized in Table 6.2.

A concept related to this research is "affect heuristic", which refers to a proposal that representations of objects and events are imbued with an emotional tone that influences judgments. A heuristic is a conventional, short-cut decision rule. An example of this heuristic is the inverse relationship between perceived risk and perceived benefit, i.e. that risk is perceived as low and benefit as high for an attractive object or target, and vice versa for unattractive ones (Finucane, Alhakami, Slovic, & Johnson, 2000).

6.3 Reason and Emotion

The results from studies which were cited in this chapter may suggest that Plato and Aristotle were wrong. Emotions are no threat to reason. It may be that reason, i.e. cognition, can be influenced by some emotions to select simplified and superficial solutions to some problems, and be influenced by other emotions to be conservative and analytical. Emotions may also lead to a focus on some part of an experience at the expense of others, and may both facilitate and hamper the memory. And, furthermore, emotions may also be the reason that something is learnt or recalled at all, which means that reason is dependent on and even presupposed by emotion. It may be reminded, as was hinted at in Chap. 1, that it is the energy which is aroused by happiness, anger, sadness, and interest which awakens our consciousness and makes us look around for solution to problems and to reason. This argumentation is supported by the neurologist Antonio Damasio (1994), who pointed out that reason (cognition) cannot function in patients with large damage to the emotional part of their brain.

6.4 Practical Relevance

Questions about evaluations and congruency are parts of daily life. We are frequently in situations where we have to evaluate if something is negative or positive, dangerous or safe or challenging, indifferent or worthy. Our evaluations are often related to experiences from when we were younger, and may be more or less adequate for the present situation. It is, for example, a common fault to evaluate all dogs as dangerous based on experiences from childhood long after one has grown up and become able to defend oneself. All these instances are relevant for results from studies cited in this chapter which showed that cognition is influenced by emotion. They point to the fact that you should be conscious of your emotions when you consider your evaluations. To what extent are they, and to what extent are you dominated by emotional variations?

There is extensive professional application of the relation between emotion and cognition. A main arena for this is the court, where people's memories and behaviors are constantly evaluated for emotional influence. Another main arena is psychotherapy, where the therapist is using a number of cognitive techniques to help change the patients' coping with painful emotional reactions. The most frequent efforts is related to changing the patients' appraisals by changing negative valences («there will always be negative consequences»), support security by counteracting images of danger and catastrophes, instructing how to make effective efforts by changes in coping, and counteracting patients' tendencies of exaggerated acceptance of responsibility for others' emotions.

6.5 Summary

Results from a pioneering study by Lazarus and Alfert showed that emotion can be the result of cognition in terms of appraisals of stimuli and events. Appraisals may be a simple sorting of something as good or bad (primary appraisal), but may be dependent on a secondary appraisal of valence (the degree of positivity/negativity), security (the degree of knowledge), effort (the degree of effort needed to reach a goal), and responsibility (the degree of responsibility or causation for an event).

Results from studies on the influence of emotion on cognition has shown marked effects of congruence, which is a concordance of emotion type and cognitive functioning in memory, attention, perception, and evaluation. The intensity of negative emotion, which has been studied mainly in relation to fear, is related to excellent recall of central information and to little recall of peripheral emotion. This has direct relevance for the evaluation of reports from witnesses to criminal events.

Results from research on positive emotions have shown that happiness is generally related to creative, flexible and deductive reasoning, but may also be related to simplified and superficial thought. Sadness has, by comparison, been related to analytic, systematic and inductive reasoning that seems to include a depressive and realistic thinking.

Reflection Questions

1. Is "congruence" an example of emotions' selective drive?
2. Effects of emotion have been related to all cognitive processes. This can support a viewpoint that emotion are always "into" cognition because there must be some emotional arousal of energy to set cognition in motion. Does that mean that thinking cannot be "neutral" or "objective"?

Research/Exercise Examples

1. Test your emotion-related memory alone or with your study-group by stimulating sadness and happiness by appropriate emotions. Arrange yourself in a relaxing position and listen to the music until you can feel the emotion in the song, rate the intensity of the emotion on a five-point scale (very low-a little-some-much-very high), and then write a short note on your memory for something written on a card. The card should be drawn from a stack where each contains a subject, such as "your first year in school", "your first memories of your parents", "your body as a youngster", "your social skills in kindergarten", and "your childhood adaptation". The card-drawing procedure is proposed to avoid that you unconsciously prepare your response in the music phase.
2. Flash-bulb memory does ordinarily refer to or common experiences, but it is also meaningful to assume that people have private flash-bulb memories, i.e. sudden, salient and very clear experiences of specific events in their life. Which is your (and your fellow students') flash-bulb memories from the private life, what were the emotions involved and what were their common characteristics?

Further Reading

Lench, H. C., Flores, S. A., & Bench, S. W. (2011). Discrete emotions predict changes in cognition, judgment, experience, behavior, and physiology: a meta-analysis of experimental emotion elicitations. *Psychological Bulletin, 137*, 834–855.

Scherer, K. R. (1993). Studying the emotion-antecedent appraisal process: An expert systems approach. In N. H. Frijda (Ed.), *Appraisal and beyond. A special issue of Cognition and Emotion* (pp. 325–356). Hillsdale, NJ: Lawrence Erlbaum.

Zajonc, R. B. (1980). Feeling and thinking: Preferences need no inferences. *American Psychologist, 35*, 151–175.

Emotions and Health

7

Teil I

This chapter is introduced with a short reference to mental health, but the chapter is focused on the relation between emotions and physical health. Physical health is directly related to the definition of emotion which relates emotional arousal to reactions on all levels in the body (see Sects. 1.2 and 1.3). The part of this chapter starts with a sketch of three central processes in the relation between emotions and health: (a) The autonomous nervous system (ANS), (b) The hypothalamus-pituitary-adrenal cortex axis (HPA axis), and (c) The immunological function in the body. This is followed by a presentation of viewpoints and discussion related to the repression of emotions as a cause of illness, and further to the diathesis-stress and stress-coping models in modern approaches to the relation between emotion and health. The last part of the chapter concerns the contribution of individual emotions and shows a marked bias in focus on fear/anxiety, sadness, and anger which also is evident in approaches to mental health.

7.1 Mental Health

Emotions have traditionally been considered as belonging to the mental area, and problems have been conceived as comprising too much, too intense and/or badly controlled negative emotions of fear, sadness, and/or anger. This has also been related to health, and emotions have for a long time, especially in the Western tradition, been conceived as disturbances both of reason and health. Prominent doctors proposed that emotions were causes of both mental and physical problems when modern medicine emerged in the seventeenth century. There was, for instance, a common notion in the eighteenth century that intense emotions ("passions") could lead to problems with the soul (Taylor, 1997b). The first classification systems of mental health problems appeared in the 19th century. Classification has since then been developed into diagnostic descriptions, and about 75% of the categories in the most comprehensive diagnostic system (DSM-V, American Psychiatric Association, 2013) consists of emotional characteristics. Sections for "mood" and "anxiety" disorders comprise, for instance, a large number of disorders with emotions as the main problem (see also Werner & Gross, 2010).

There is much variation in roles attributed to emotions in mental health problems. In addition to being seen as- or indicating-problems because of their intense, frequent and/or unusual expression, emotions are conceived as an intrinsic parts of a problem (e.g. in schizophrenia), as part of the causes of the problems (e.g. the lack of guilt and the high threshold for fear in psychopathy), and as indirect causes and/or effects related to other factors, such as personality traits, traumatic childhood experiences or loss of a loved person. Emotions are even seen as involved in health problems because they are not accessed by a person's consciousness, such as Sally in Table 1.1, and as persons suffering from alexithymia, i.e. the lack of ability to use words for emotions.

The overwhelming majority of emotions related to mental health problems are fear, sadness, and anger. Guilt has been discussed in relation to psychoneurosis, and shame, which was noted in Sect. 3.2.2 as a domineering force of several cultures was largely ignored in mental health research before the 1990s (Tangney, 1995). Envy, analyzed by Schoeck (Schoeck, 1969) as a main driver of human behavior and political ideologies, and depicted together with jealousy by screenwriters and novelists for their invasive effects on persons' mental life seem to be completely ignored. Happiness, which may be the focused emotion by the general public, has likewise been ignored but may be on its way to recognition in the wake of modern research on positive emotions (see Sect. 3.1).

The fear-sadness-aggression bias in studies and discussions of emotions' influence on mental health leads to an ignorance of the influence from individual emotions and of effects of interactions and blends of emotions. Examples of interaction may be that sadness can be increased by low access to happiness, and that aggression may be increased or inhibited by fear. An example of blending may be the combination of anger, disgust, and contempt evident in the hostility which is a salient characteristic of the "Dark Triad" of narcissism, Machiavellianism, and psychopathy (Izard, 1972).

The vast literature on emotions in mental health cannot be referred in the present book. One reason is that the mental health area lacks objective and independent indications of when a person has a mental health problem. There is no objective indicator of mental health which parallels the physiological indicators (blood pressure, temperature, etc.) of health in physiological functioning. It is therefore, for instance, difficult

A. Vikan, *A Fast Road to the Study of Emotions*,
DOI 10.1007/978-3-319-52313-2_7

to differentiate indication of health problems from "normal", or even "healthy" aggressive or anxious responses when the environment is threatening in some way. Another reason is that there exists no definition of healthy emotional functioning. A third reason for excluding reference of the literature on mental health that studies have been conducted within different professions (medicine, psychology, social work) without a commonly accepted definition of emotion. "Emotion" in psychiatric research is, for instance, often called "affect", and may refer both to physiological processes and expressive behavior, whereas "emotion" in clinical psychology refers to cognition and is based on patients' self-reports and responses to interviews. This hampers the building of scientific evidence because comparisons of results are often not possible.

7.2 Physical Health

Physical health is directly related to the definition of emotion which relates emotional arousal to reactions on all levels in the body (Sects. 1.2 and 1.3). A dramatic example of this relatedness is probably that sudden and extreme emotional arousal may lead to heart failure and death (Wittstein et al., 2005). This demonstrates that emotional processes are part of the integrated, balanced state of the organism and its adaptation to the environment which is referred to by the concept of health. Studies in the area started late in the 20th century, and have not lacked aims and targets after the realization that emotions is at the core of social illness. Social illness refers to health problems with a background in the social- and interpersonal aims as related to efforts to obtain an education, anxieties regarding the obligations at the workplace, worries about loans and other responsibilities, and conflicts involving anger, insecurity, and sadness related to wishes, expectations, and duties in the family. A common word for these emotional challenges is stress. Illnesses and nuisances which have been related to stress are cardiovascular problems, psychosomatic illness, pains caused by muscular problems, diabetes, ulcer, obesity and drug dependency. This can indicate that social illnesses, together with mental health problems and cancer, are modern society's most extensive and expensive problems. Emotions are *the* problem in mental health, and as they have also been related to cancer (Reiche, Morimoto, & Nunes, 2006), it may seem that emotions are the key to the prevention and treatment of a population's health problems.

7.3 Three Systems in the Body's Response to Emotional Stress

Three systems are especially involved in emotional arousal: The Autonomous Nervous System (ANS), the HPA-axis, and the Immune System. The resulting extent of these is that the whole body, from the nails and the skin to the blood, the intestines, the brain stem and several areas of the brain itself functions as a kind of a tuning fork for emotions. It may also be proposed that the relation between emotions and the body's physiological functions is so close and reciprocal that physiological reactions may be conceived as emotional expressions.

The autonomous nervous system (ANS). The ANS constitutes, together with the somatic nervous system, a system which is «peripheral» by registering stimulation from the outer (toes and fingers) to the inner (the intestines) parts of the body. ANS consists of the sympathic and the parasympathic system with reciprocally balancing functions as is indicated in Table 7.1.

Table 7.1 The distribution of functions in the ANS

Sympathic system
Increases blood pressure, pulse, and sweating
Increases blood sugar, velocity of the blood stream and oxygen absorption
Decreases spit, slime and gastrointestinal mobility
Reroutes blood from the intestines to the brain and the skeletal muscles
Parasympathic system
Directs the digestion
Maintains the body's resources
Decreases blood pressure, pulse, breathing, etc.
Reacts generally contrary to sympathetic activation

The nerves in ANS end in the smooth muscles in the vascular system, the heart, the inner organs in general and the sweat glands. When the brain receives sensations which are registered as important, for instance in terms of an emotion, it sends a message about measures which must be initiated by activity in the sympathetic system. One of the measures is noradrenaline, a transmitter substance which influences the transmission of nerve impulses, stimulates the secretion of the hormone adrenaline from the adrenal gland, and serves to activate the whole ANS in seconds.

The HPA-axis. The HPA-axis is a pattern of stimulation from the brain to the adrenal gland. Frequent emotional arousal activates reactions in the hypothalamus, which is an area located centrally in the brain (see Figs. 1.6 and 12.2). Hormonal secretion in the hypothalamus stimulates hormonal activity in the pituitary, which is a gland at the underside of the brain. These hormones relate messages to the adrenal gland located at the top of the kidneys. The adrenal gland secretes cortisol, which is known as a "stress hormone". Cortisol stimulates to increase in the production of blood sugar, which increases the body' energy, but suppresses at the same time the functioning of the immune system. The activity along the HPA-axis is represented in Fig. 7.1. (see page 51).

The immune systemet. The immune system is often called the «immune defense» because the system's main function is to reject and/or destroy invaders (virus, bacteria) in the body. The system affects and is affected by the nervous system by transmitter substances at the nerve endings. This shows that what is registered as an emotional strain in the brain also

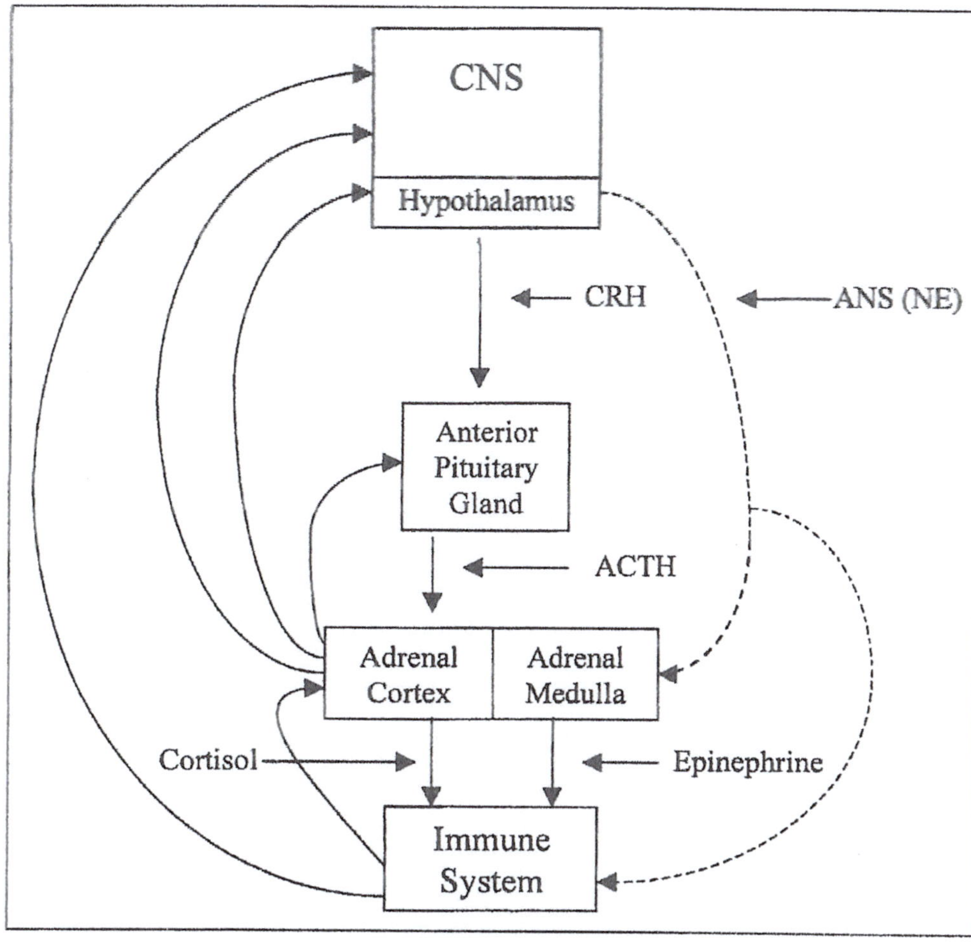

Fig. 7.1 Schematic representation of the HPA-axis which shows interrelationships among the central nervous system (CNS), the hypothalamic-pituitary-adrenal axis, the ANS and the immune system. *Dashed lines* indicate ANS neural pathways, *solid lines* indicate hormonal pathways. *ACT* adrenocorticotropic hormone; *CHR* cortocotropic-releasing hormone; *NE* norepinephrine (from Kemeny, 2003)

affects the immune system. This influence results generally in a weakening of the immune system which makes the body more vulnerable to illness.

The immune system comprises white blood cells which are circulated in the blood- and lymphatic system. It is in two main parts: Fagocytes, which is formed in the bone marrow, and lymphocytes, which is formed in the spleen and lympathic nodes. The function of the fagocytes is to release immune responses by way of cytokines (e.g. the peptid homone PIC), which call in assistance when there is a virus attack. The lymphocytes consist of B- and T-cells. The T-cells kills microorganisms and releases the B-cells, which produces antibodies which «remembers» invaders to secure a quicker response to the next attack. One type of cells is called "natural killers", or "NK-cells", and is directed at killing invaders. See examples in Table 7.3 (see page 55) of immune system responses in relation to individual emotions.

Porges (2011) have argued that there is a third, polyvagal system related to the vagus nerve with parasympathetic effects which is central to the regulation of emotional arousal. The function and consequences of this is not sufficiently established for a further presentation here.

7.4 Repression and the Question Whether Emotions Should Be Suppressed or Displayed Openly

It is evident from the preceding section that emotions are related to physiological processes which are central to the body's health. This is the backbone of the "social illness" concept that factors which affect emotions also affect health. It means that emotion is a variable which mediates the effects of environmental factors on the physiological processes which determine health. This has not always been realized in discussions where emotions are related to health by association to environmental- (threats, demands) and physiological variables (illness, hypersensitivity), which are easily measured and have been focused in research.

Emotions are focused when it is realized that neither challenging environments nor vulnerable physiology leads automatically to health problems but relates to persons' (subjective) emotional response. And as emotions are common human qualities it can be assumed that health problems are related to

Table 7.2 Models for the relation between emotions and health problems

Psychoanalysis (from 1930-1940) Inner conflicts ↓ Repressed emotions ↓ Compromises between drives and social norms ↓ Psychosomatic illness	**Engel-Schmale-Eysenck (about 1980)** Tension of negative emotions and lack of personal independence ↓ Helplessness, hopelessness and shame reactions ↓ Cancer
Glover-MacAlpine (1940-1950) Primitive, partly expressed emotions not articulated in language ↓ Problems of expressing and understanding emotions ↓ Psychosomatic illness	**Pennebaker (1990)** Emotional tension ↓ Inhibiting emotional expression ↓ Physiological work which weaken the immune system ↓ Physical illness
Sifneos (1970-1980) Large problems in verbal expressions of emotions (alexithymia) ↓ Increased vulnerability for illness ↓ Psychosomatic- and other illnessess	**Taylor (1997a)** Integrated model ↓ Emotional tension ↓ Wrongful regulation of ANS-neuroendocrinological activation ↓ Physical illness

Based on Taylor (1997a)

the manner in which persons handle their emotions. The discussion on this point has been inspired Freud's psychoanalytic theory and the concept of repression in the 1890s. Repression refers to a more or less conscious "expulsion" of drives (sexuality and aggression) and emotional experiences from consciousness. The concept was established when Freud discovered that mental problems of his patients were associated with childhood experiences which the patients were not able to recall before they were assisted and help by Freud's free association method. The patients' "forgetting" was interpreted as a repression which results in memories which continue to influence persons functioning in ways that hampered their health and adaptation.

The bridge between the mental repression mechanism and physical health was explicitly realized by the psychoanalyst Alexander (1939, 1950), who pointed to repressed emotions as the major cause of psychosomatic illness. Alexander's theories were presented in 1930–1940, and have inspired several models for how health problems relate to emotions which are repressed, suppressed (the conscious variant of repression), are difficult to express and/or are regulated in dysfunctional ways. An overview over the best known models is shown in Table 7.2.

All models in Table 7.2 imply that emotional factors contribute with other factors in processes which lead to illness. Repression or similar consequences (lack of adequate expression of emotion) are assumed in four of the models to be direct causes of illnesses. All models imply that inadequate emotional expression is harmful to health.

Studies on repression has been conducted by using scales with items in terms of questions to which degree the respondent would like to forget, overlook, or not mind an unpleasant experience. Such scales have often been used together with a corresponding scale for openness as a control for the consistence of responses. Items in openness scales are about the degree to which the respondent will examine the experience and causes of an emotion. Each scale may consist of 10–20 items, and each response is allocated a point from 0–4 corresponding to the rating on a five-point scale from «very much» to «not at all».

This measurement means, according to the repression concept, that persons with health problems score high on a repression scale and low on an openness scale, whereas persons without health problems show the opposite pattern of scores. Examples of such scales are "repression versus sensitization" (Byrne, 1961), "blunting versus monitoring" (Miller, 1987) and "avoidance versus vigilance" (Krohne, Hock, & Kohlmann, 1992).

The results from studies with the scales have not been unequivocal. There is robust documentation that persons with high scores on repression scales are more often ill than persons with low scores (Myers & Derakshan, 2004), and that there is an association between repression of negative emotions, cardiovascular disease and hypertension (Mauss & Gross, 2004) . But the evidence is also robust that emotional arousal leads to wear and tear and health problems. Persons who blunt (repress) information seem, for instance, to maintain a low emotional tension, while those who monitor the information do that at the cost of a high level of tension (Miller, 1987). The results of these studies can, therefore, not be a convincing answer to whether emotions or their expressions should be suppressed. Other studies seem, unfortunately, also to provide divided evidence on the question.

Emotions should be expressed openly. Support from openness is primarily related to a series of studies which were initiated by Pennebaker and Beall (1986). The study began with an invitation to college-students to write about negative events in their lives that they had never talked to anybody about. They responded to health questionnaires and were tested with physiological measures before the writing and some months afterwards. The results, which were supported by results from several subsequent studies, showed that the writing lead to a decrease in somatic problems, and to less frequent visit to medical doctors. The students also showed an increase in immune functioning and a decrease in mental problems. Pennebaker (1989, 1990) assumed that writing loosened the repressive inhibitions on the memory and freed energy which had been used to hide their mental wounds. The new energy was assumed to be used to strengthen the immune defense, which were weakened while the inhibition was in place (see the model of Pennebaker's theory in Table 7.2).

Pennebaker's inhibition theory was weakened by results from later studies which have shown that writing about recently experienced and current problems have parallel effects to writing about events many years ago (Greenberg & Lepore, 2004). It has even been suggested that writing about fantasized traumas have resulted in positive effects on health (Greenberg, Wortman, & Stone, 1996). Although these results may be critical to the inhibition interpretation, they may still seem to support the assumption that emotional expression, at least in writing, is positive for health.

Emotions should be suppressed (controlled). Part of the evidence for healthy effects of suppression will be referred to in Sect. 7.5, where it is noted that «free flow» of anger and hostility may lead to cardiovascular problems. This may mean that a question about suppression should be related to emotion types. An assumption may be that anger is best suppressed, while fear and sadness should be expressed openly. Contrary evidence is that sadness has been shown to result in worry and rumination which worsens the problem (Nolen-Hoeksema, McBride, & Larson, 1997). Another example of this is perseverative thinking, which means a circling around the same negative theme in a worried and ruminating way. This type of ruminative repetitions is often part of anxiety problems.

These contradictory results may mean that the dimension of control of emotions, which is represented by the variation from repression/suppression to openness, is not sufficient and may be too simple, to describe how handling of emotions is related to health. An alternative model was suggested from Walter Cannon's studies in the 1920s on crisis reactions in rats, and was developed by use of the concepts of stress and coping.

7.5 Stress, Emotion, and Health

Cannon (1927) showed that what he called fear and anger in rats were parts of crisis reactions of, respectively, flight or attack performed with energy which was mobilized via the ANS. Selye (1956) extended this to a three-phase model which may represent how emotions lead to health problems. Phase 1 consists of alarm reactions which trigger the mobilization of energy resources in the body. Phase 2 is a resistance phase which consists of the use of different types of coping. Phase 3 is an exhaustion phase where the energy is spent and the resistance has collapsed. Selye used the concept of stress for the mobilization of resources, and the word "stressor" to denote the straining and challenging stimulation or event which triggers stress reactions.

The concept of stress directed the attention to reactions to stressors. Analyses of physiological responses led to the insight that physical health problems are related to life- and/or work situations where the main stressors are emotional. Results from studies of stress reactions have suggested that stress may result in the serious illnesses noted in the introduction to the chapter (see update in Anisman, 2014), in addition to several other types of problems, such as dwarfism and analgesia (Sapolsky, 1994). The problem for research on stress is the "subjectivity factor" which was noted in the introduction to Sect. 7.3, and which refers to the fact that stress relates to individual perception and experience. Failure at an exam or the loss of a close friend is, for instance, stressing for most students, but not for all. A health problem may therefore be a question both of persons' individual make-up and stressors from the environment. This is built into the diathesis-stress model, which is one of two prominent models in the area.

Diathesis-stress is a model is related to a conception that health problems are the result of an interaction of predispositions or vulnerabilities (diathesis) and environmental stressors. Vulnerabilities are genetic deviation or biologically based weakness, and the model represents an insight that health problems is often the consequence of a point in an interaction rather than one specific cause of some kind. This means, for instance, that vulnerability or weakness only becomes part of an illness in relation to some, but not all types of environmental stress. And, conversely, that environmental stress only results in illness for some, i.e. those with a specific vulnerability, but not all persons. Emotion has been entered in the model as vulnerabilities in general terms of "impulsivity", "hostility", and "anxiousness", and diathesis-stress has been useful in analyses of mental health problems such as schizophrenia (e.g. Yank, Bentley, & Hargrove, 1993) and depression (e.g. Pardilla, & Calvete, 2015).

The other model in the area is the stress-coping paradigm. The central concept is "coping", which refers to conscious efforts to handle, tolerate, or reduce stressful challenges in the environment. Health in this context is a question of how a person copes with environmental stressors rather than a question of suppression or expression of emotions. The paradigm was initiated in the 1980s, and was rapidly adopted by researchers who discovered that they met with parallel problems in finding measures of stress and coping. Aldwin (1994) noted, for instance, that there were 82 different methods of measuring coping, and more that 2000 published articles and books on stress already in the five years 1988–1993. The reason for the large number on coping is that coping depends on persons' development and competence, and will, consequently, be different for children, adolescents, adults, and older people. Coping will also vary with problem type and situation, and measures must, therefore, be related to variations in situations for each sample. The same instrument is, e.g. not appropriate in coping with divorce, traffic accident and illnesses such as diabetes and cancer.

The best known and most frequently employed measure of coping is "The Ways of Coping Checklist" (WCC) (Folkman & Lazarus, 1980). The check-list consists of 68 measures which are rated on four-point scales from"do not use" to"uses frequently" in relation to a personally experienced stressful situation that the person is asked to imagine. Lazarus and co-workers identified two general dimensions in coping: Problem-focused and emotion-focused coping, which refer to, respectively, attempts to solve the problem which has emerged or attempts to handle one's emotions in the situation. Examples of problem-focused coping are: "Made a plan and followed it","fetched help from an expert", and "analyzed the problem to understand it in a better way". Examples of emotion-focused coping are: "Behave as if nothing has happened", "pray to God", and "talk to somebody about my emotions". A third general dimension of avoidance, comprising a tendency to cope by seeking out other people (social diversion) and/or by engaging in substitute tasks (distraction) has been identified by Endler and Parker (1994).

A large number of studies have convincingly shown that coping is related to health. Problem-focused coping has, for instance, been associated with less mental and physical health problems than emotion-focused coping, but this also seems to be related to types of situations. Problem-focused coping and openness may, generally, be preferable in situations where persons have some control and possibility of action, whereas emotion-focused coping and suppression may be preferable (and often the only possible coping) in situations with very little or no control. Results from studies on coping have in addition been very useful for information and prevention of health and for preparation of medical compliance and treatment both outside and inside the hospitals.

It may not be possible to overstate the significance of the enormous and widely influential area of stress research on the understanding of health, but the relation to emotions may seem paradoxical: Emotions are always present and shown as influences on health at the same time as they are practically invisible. This is because "stress" comprises an undifferentiated sample of emotions and includes other processes (i.e. attention, problem-solving, social interaction). There is, undoubtedly, still much to be learnt from studies of stress when the contribution from individual emotions can be distinguished. Lazarus (1993, p. 10) referred to this when he stated that "…recognition of 15 or so specific emotions instead of several dimensions of stress greatly increases what we can say about individual's coping and adaptation".

7.6 Effect of Individual Emotions on Physiological Processes and Health

The main interest on the relation between emotions and health from the perspective of emotions is if and how health is related to individual emotions. This has scarcely been considered in research on stress and coping, which has mainly been related to emotions in terms of a general factor of negative emotions. A promising breakthrough for insight into the effect on health of specific emotions was the medical doctors Friedman and Roseman's (1974) description of Type-A personality in the 1960–1970s. Type-A personality refers to a person who is characterized as impatient, irritable, aggressive, and dominant. Friedman and Roseman's discovery was that this type of personality was very frequent among their patients with infarct. Results from subsequent studies have confirmed that there is a clear association of Type-A personality and cardiovascular problems. Type-A has also been described as an "AHA-syndrome" comprised by anger, hostility, and aggression (Johnson, 1990; Mauss & Gross, 2004) .

The promise of the discovery of the Type-A personality has not been fulfilled. Other clear connections between an individual emotion (anger) and specific health problems have not been identified. A proposal of an association of a Type-B relaxed and «mild» personality with a tendency of depression and associated with cancer has not been convincingly supported by research. A main problem in this context is that the concept and measurement of stress refers to a general activation of negative emotions (fear/anxiety, anger, sadness, shame, and guilt). This fails to identify contributions from individual emotions which may be responsible for problems in health. This point is supported by results from emotion regulation studies which have shown that individual emotions may be regulated in different ways (Rivers, Brackett, Katulac, & Salovey, 2007; Vikan, Rugseth, & Hassel, 2010).

Some evidence pertaining to individual emotions do exist. Kemeny and Shestyuk (2008) have reviewed the evidence of health effects associated with individual emotions. Health effects in this context refer to how an emotion may influence

Table 7.3 Oversight of effects of individual emotions on health

Anger and hostility
AHA-syndrome connected with increase in blood-pressure, infarct and increased mortality and mortality risk, and increased activation and weakened inhibition in hypothalamus because of low access to serotonin
AHA-persons show peripheral inflammation because of increased PIC which indicates arteriosclerosis and infarct
Hostility related to increase in colesterol and simulation of inflammation leading to weakened immune functioning because of less ability to breed immune cells in addition to decrease in NK-cells
Fear and anxiety
Increased risk of cardiovascular illness because of activation of noradrenaline. Increased activation of HPA-axis and secretion of cortisol
Decreased immune functioning (NK-cell activity) related to increase in Anxiety because of disturbance of formation of interleukin-2 cytokines
Negative affect and depression
Insufficient serotonin and dopamine (which stimulate positive emotions) HPA dysregulation and increased secretion of cortisol
Asymmetric electrical activity in the brain which can relate to lower immunoglobulin after flu vaccination, and to lower NK cell activity
Decreased immune function in terms of decrease in B and T cells and activity in NK-cells, increased levels and/or increased production of PIC
Shame
Shame-situations activate HPA and secrete cortisol
Indications of higher production of PIC
Positive emotions
Generally better health
Increase in frontal left-hemisphere asymmetry and in activation of serotonin, dopamin and noradrenaline with inhibition of HPA-activation
Increased secretory immunoglobin A, which increases lymphocytic breeding response and NK cells

Based on Kemeny and Shestyuk (2008)

processes which are relevant for health. An overview of results from research is provided in Table 7.3. Kemeny and Shestyuk concluded their review by writing (2008, p. 671): "There is increasing evidence that affective experiences are associated with important changes in peripheral regulatory systems intimately tied to health and disease".

It may be assumed that the problems noted in Table 7.3 result in illness depending on the frequency, intensity, and duration of the arousal of an emotion. Table 7.3 shows a focus on fear/anxiety, anger, and sadness similar to the bias of emotions in mental health. The focus on shame and positive emotions are more recent, while consequences of interest, disgust, surprise, contempt, and guilt has not been studied at all. It should, moreover, be noted that studies on anxiety and sadness has been related to persons with psychiatric diagnoses. This might mean that the effect of several emotions are blended because persons with problem diagnoses of one of these emotions often have problems with the other, and both may be related to shame (Vikan, Johnsen, Moen, Hassel, & Rugseth, 2010). Psychiatric diagnoses may also involve specific behaviors (e.g. much passivity) which have health effects that may be confounded with effects from the emotions themselves. There is, therefore, a high degree of uncertainty related to the effects shown in Table 7.3. It also remains a large and open question whether different emotions have effects that reinforce or counteract each other.

7.7 Practical Relevance

The results in Chap. 6 that emotions are influenced by cognition represent an entrance to the practical relevance of the relation between emotion and health in this chapter. In fact, the effect of cognition on emotion, the association of emotions and physiological processes, and the effects of physiological processes on health suggest a causal sequence as the one in Fig. 7.2.

The model implies an assumption that a person's health is determined by a person's own cognition and her/his ways of regulating emotions. The model also suggests that schools and workplaces may be environments which might be prepared to stimulate healthy emotional experiences. Several techniques have been developed within cognitive psychotherapy to identify and replace unhealthy cognitions of emotions.

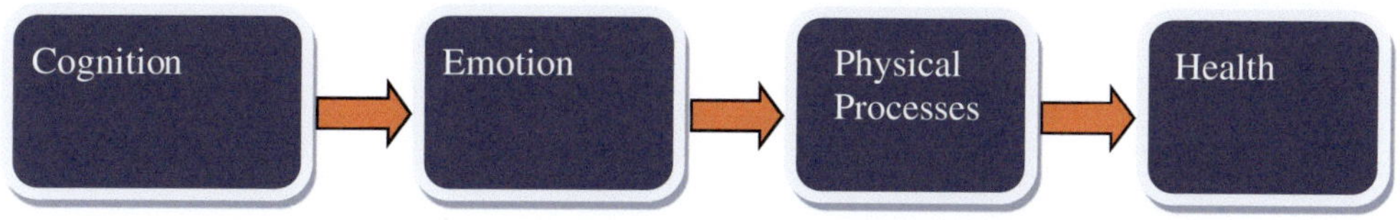

Fig. 7.2 Causal sequence from cognition through emotion to health

Strategies for healthy strategies are indicated in the next chapter (Chap. 8).

Practical relevance is often shown in many campaigns for health-related information from central governments and health institutions. Specific adjustments, for example in preparing children for medical treatment, have also been based on experiences from studies on emotions' effect on health.

7.8 Summary

Emotions have been realized as source of cardiovascular problems, psychosomatic illness, pains related to muscular problems, diabetes, ulcer, obesity and drug dependency, which also have been conceived as social illnesses. Emotions influence health mainly via the ANS, the HPA-axis and the immune system.

The cause of emotional problems was first conceived as repressions. Studies related to this concept have resulted in contradictory results. Pennebaker and co-workers showed that writing about negative experienced which had never been shared with others resulted in several indications of improved health, while studies of openly and frequently displayed aggression and hostility in A-type and AHA-type personality was clearly related to cardiovascular illness, and that expression of anxiety and sadness in terms of, respectively, worry and rumination also was related to negative health indices.

Most studies on the relation between emotion and help has been based on concepts of stress and coping. Coping has been differentiated into the three basic dimensions: Problem-focused, emotion-focused and avoidance oriented coping, and results have indicated that problem-focused coping is associated with better measures of health than the emotion-focused variety. The limitation of the stress-coping paradigm is that studies have been related to general measures of negative emotionality and have generally ignored the contribution of individual emotions. The health factors which have been related to individual emotions are shown in an oversight in Table 7.3.

Reflection Questions

1. Emotional factors contribute to health problems mostly as long term effects, and are difficult to identify. Responses which are comparatively immediate and direct are asthmatic reactions, chest pain (angina), migraine, tensed muscles (especially in the jaw, neck, and upper arms), eczema reactions, loss of sleep, loss of appetite, and stomach pains. Do you recognize instances of these responses from events in your life, and can you relate them to emotional events which may have triggered them?
2. What coping strategies do you and your fellow students use, and in what way to you use them? Do you use coping strategies independent of the emotion involved (i.e. do you use emotion-focused coping both for anger and fear)?

Research/Exercise Examples

1. Medical doctors often find it difficult to convince patients that their illness is related to emotions and stress. Design a study to explore to what extent people, differentiated by gender, age, and education, think that there is a relation between health and stress, one the one hand, and health and emotions on the other.
2. Physiotherapists can generally relate many examples of emotional reactions, mostly sadness/crying or anger, when they start massaging tensed muscles. You can test your own responses, and therefore also emotional investments in your body, by having your muscles in the face (especially the forehead, chins and jaw) and neck slowly and sensitively massaged, and noting the emotional responses related directly to the touch as well as those which seem to function as avoidance of contact.

Further Reading

DeSteno, D., Gross, J. J., & Kubansky, L. (2013). Affective science and health: The importance of emotion and emotion regulation. *Health Psychology, 32,* 474–486.

Lazarus, R. S. (1993). From psychological stress to the emotions: A history of changing outlooks. *Annual Review of Psychology, 44,* 1–21.

Nyklicek, I., Temoshok, L., & Vingerhoets, A. (Eds.) (2004). *Emotional expression and health*. New York: Brunner–Routledge.

Emotion Regulation

8

Teil I

There have been several references in this book to the fact that emotions can be handled, mastered, controlled, coped with, repressed or regulated. The generic term in modern research for these phenomena is «emotion regulation». This chapter starts with a short presentation of the concept of emotion regulation, and is continued with a description of emotion regulation at birth and in the child's first and second year and proceeds to description of the first verbal strategies, such as stop being sad, angry, or afraid in the child's fourth year. A main task for new research in an area is to establish an overview. This chapter, therefore, comprises a description of three approaches to the classification of manners or strategies for emotion regulation. The approaches are Hochschildt's (1979) theory on emotion rules and emotion work, Gross' (1998, 2002; Gross & Thompson, 2007) model for components in emotion regulation, and Parkinson and Totterdell's (1999) classification of emotion regulation strategies.

8.1 The Concept of Emotion Regulation

Emotion regulation may consist of counting to ten as a distraction from anger, eating to suppress sadness, or select some music to obtain a happy feeling. The concept has been defined as « the processes involved in modifying emotional reactions » (Oatley & Jenkins, 1996, p. 192), and as "extrinsic and intrinsic processes" that « …subdue (or enhance) the intensity of expressed emotion, retard (or speed) its onset or recovery, limit (or enhance) its persistence over time, reduce (or increase) emotion range or lability, and affect other qualitative features of emotions responding (Thompson, 1994, p. 29). The target of emotion regulation is initiatives pertaining to specific emotions and/or emotional intensity. Notice that this is different from the target of the stress and coping paradigm which was the adaptation in challenging situations that elicited a blend of negative emotional reactions.

Research on emotion regulation is comparatively recent. An open search on the PsycInfo 01.02.2016 showed, for instance, that 83.2% (n = 10,448) of articles and books on emotion regulation were published in 2005–2015, as compared to 6.2% in 1990–2000.

8.2 Development of Emotion Regulation

Emotion regulation was first used as a concept to describe the behavior of infants and young children. This was related to studies of infants' temperaments which showed that some children were "open" and adapted easily to stimulation, while others were comparatively "closed" and needed a slow habituation (Derryberry & Rothbart, 1997). This was interpreted as different ways of regulating tension. Regulation was conceived as motivated by the need to maintain an inner, organismic balance (homeostasis). Tension was conceived as an indication of emotion, and the first reflexive reactions were, accordingly, conceived as ways of regulating emotions. The most "radical" reaction of this type is that infants may go into sleep as a response to intense and sudden stimulation. Common tension-reducing reactions indicated by infants is turning of the head, disengagement of visual attention (look another way), and stopping breathing and crying (Kopp & Neufeldt, 2003).

The first regulations are inherited mechanisms that secures a balance in the body' functioning. They contribute to modulate the senses' information absorption in relation to other functions such as sleep, appetite or digestion. This is a demonstration of emotion regulation's biological anchoring and cooperation with other processes in the body, and shows that it is affected and affects biological processes.

Regulation is influenced by social interaction a short time after birth when the infant is awake for longer periods and able to record stimulation from the surroundings. The child will for more than a year from about three months after birth be dependent on interaction with CP as support for their emotional regulation (Sroufe, 1996). Table 8.1 (see page 58) comprises an overview of regulation types in this age period, and indicates regulation adapted from the interaction in terms of active avoidance, orientation towards CP, approach and attack. These are used together reflexive mechanisms related to attention and breathing.

A. Vikan, *A Fast Road to the Study of Emotions*,
DOI 10.1007/978-3-319-52313-2_8

The influence from interactions with CP results in relatively stable emotional patterns of attachment at about seven months of age. The 65–70% of children whose CP read their emotional signals and adjust to their needs have been shown as open and trusting in their emotional expressions. 10–15% of children whose CP is characterized by rigid rules and lack of accept of emotions have been observed to over-regulate and show few emotional expressions. Another 10–15% of children have been observed to under-regulate and show labile and intense emotional reactions and be related to CPs characterized by sudden variations between openness and lack of access, and between permissiveness and rigid rules. A fourth pattern has been described as an emotional chaos in children without a stable and caring CP. The patterns have been shown to be stable until adulthood, but they may change with changes in the family and environment, and are also influenced by cultural patterns (van Ijzendoorn & Sagi-Schwartz, 2008).

The development of the self from the middle of the second year is a first and not very robust foundation of the child's independence, and he/she will continue to depend on support and guidance from CP. The increased independence and the need for guidance is also indicated by a marked increase in cognitive and linguistic development. An overview of regulation strategies in two-year old children in Table 8.2 shows examples of cognitive regulations (strategies 1, 3 and partly 6), dependency of CP (strategies 5 and partly 6), as well as regulations from a younger age (strategies 2 and 4). The descriptions in Tables 8.1 and 8.2 are based on observations of children's actual emotion regulation.

The two year old child is also beginning to regulate her/his emotion in relation to what is morally right and wrong, and what is correct and not correct in terms of standards for behavior. This comprises a learning of social causes of positive and negative emotions, and a learning of how emotions should be expressed in different social situations. The child internalizes this learning as a set of values between the ages two and four. This becomes part of a steering system which reinforces an independent foundation of emotion regulation. An example of this is that the child can begin to verbalize some regulation strategies. Thus, three-four year old children can have several propositions of what they might do to stop or become less angry, afraid, or sad. This can be propositions of social strategies («Go to mother», «Tell it to somebody»), change in the situation («By a new ball», «Turn on the light») or simply play. Some children may also propose cognitive strategies, such as: «Forget it», and «Do not think about it» (Dias, Vikan, & Gravås, 2000; Vikan, Kårstad, & Dias, 2013).

Table 8.1 Emotion regulation methods in 3–13 month old children

Active avoidance
Orientation to the caring person (CP)
Distracted attention
Approach
Attack
Movement to stimulate the body
Respiration
Self-comfort with stimulation of the skin

Based on Rothbart, Ziaie & O'Boyle (1992)

Table 8.2 Strategies for the regulation of emotion in two year old children

1. Activity with substitute toy
The child focuses on and begins to play with toys alone or with others
2. Passive use of objects and exploration
The child looks around, touches objects with the hands and looks around without active engagement
3. Symbolic self-comforting
Behavior or proposals which suggest comfort (say or thinks: "I am a big girl", "mother comes soon")
4. Physical self-comfort
Behavior directed toward the body, such as stroking one's body, twisting one's hair, and hug a teddy-bear)
5. Other-directed behavior
Seeking comfort (wanting to be held), touching an adult's hair, body, or clothes, crawling on to the lap
6. Focus on what the child is waiting for
Looking at an object, frequent questions about mother

From Grolnick, Bridges & Connell (1996)

8.3 Why Is Emotions Regulated? Feeling Rules and Emotional Work

A development of infants' need to maintain an organismic balance may be attempts to emotions in order to obtain an optimal intensity level (see Sect. 4.3) or keep a person well organized and in an emotional balance. These are organic- or inner causes of emotion regulation. Another type of causes was suggested by the description in Sect. 4.5 that emotions may be feared because they do not seem socially appropriate. This fear relates an outer, normative cause of emotion regulation. «Normative» refers to a norm, i.e. what is «usual», «appropriate», and/or «normal». The norm has an inbuilt prescription. It is something that ought to be adhered to, a rule that something should be followed. The rule has moral implications by indicating that it is morally wrong not to comply with the norm. The morality reinforces the norm with a power to act on behalf of society. This is because the rule is an instruction of how individuals shall feel and behave in a way which is similar to the instructions for roles in screenplays.

Hochschild (1979) based her influential view on emotions on assumptions that a society has norms for emotions in terms of «feeling rules» which prescribe how persons ought to feel and to express their emotions in social situation. These rules are known in terms of general statements about which emotions which can or ought to be expressed, and are also referred to as "display rules". Examples are: "You have no right to be jealous since we agreed that …", «you should rather be glad than angry when he tried to help you with …». Statements also pertain to the intensity of emotions, such as: «You must be more happy when …», and: «There is no reason to be so afraid for something as little as …», and to the duration of emotions, such as for instance: "You should be though grieving over her by now…". The examples show that feeling rules concern the relation between stimulation/events and emotional responses, and may be rather explicit as regard which emotions should be connected to specific situations. An example is that persons ought to be happy in weddings and sad in funerals. Feeling rules are also differentiated in relation to gender. Anger is, for instance, more accepted in men than in women, and in relation to social roles (a priest should always remain well controlled while a guard may be openly angry).

There is no punishment for not complying with the rules, but they have consequences by providing social "tests" which may have negative outcomes. The manner in which feeling rules is followed is a central part of the attribution of personal qualities such as "dependable", "impulsive", "egoistical", "empathic", "ruthless", or "stupid". The test may according to this engender motivation for regulating emotion in order to comply with the norm.

Hochschild referred to the effort which is necessary for regulation as «emotion work» and described two types of work, surface and depth acting. These two types can be considered as general emotion regulation strategies. *Surface acting* is focused on the outward behavior and comprises the use of gestures and behavior to form or imitate an appropriate emotion. *Deep acting* is attempts to actually feel the emotion which is acted by "psyching" oneself into the emotion. This entails to use one's imaginations and memory to induce oneself into an emotional state to the extent of believing that one actually feel the emotion in question.

8.4 James J. Gross' Model of Emotion Regulation

A new area is often best approached, as was noted in the introduction to the chapter, by questions about which types can be distinguished and how each of them functions. James J. Gross answered these questions by an overview shown in Table 8.3, and by studies which show that emotion regulation affects all components of an emotion (Gross, 2002) Gross has supported appraisal theory (see Sect. 6.2) in his view on the causation of emotions.

The upper part of the model is a sketch of a sequence of events which starts with an emotionally arousing situation, continues with the attention to the situation an appraisal of what it means, and leads to an emotion by engendering emotional reaction tendencies which are followed by a full emotional response. The sequence is a more detailed sketch of the emotional end of causation than the one in Sect. 1.6 because of Gross' differentiation between "reaction tendencies" and "emotional response". The latter refer to the actual regulation, and «reaction tendencies» refers to a holding of the emotion before it is expressed in a suitable or effective way in behavior. The concept is central to the concept of «action readiness», which is used by many authors (e.g. Frijda, 2007), and which refers to a view that emotion is always related to behavior (see Sect. 1.2).

The main point in Gross' model is that the regulation of emotions can be initiated at different points in the sequence. This is represented in the lower part of Table 8.3, which indicates that emotion regulation can be take place before the emotion is aroused (antecedent regulation focus) and before it is expressed (reaction-based regulation focus). There can be four types of antecedent- and one type reaction-based regulation strategies (Gross & Thompson, 2007). Two antecedent strategies are directed towards the selection and change of situations, which also serve as an example of how behavior is motivated by emotions (see also Sect. 1.5). Selection of situations refers to persons' strategies of avoiding situations which they know or suspect may lead to anxiety, experience of loss or failure, or to provocation which may lead, respectively, to sadness or anger, or to seek situations which they knew can make them happy, proud, or interested. Strategies related to the situation are behaviors that may change a situation, such as turning off a TV if the program is disturbing, or ask for pardon for a behavior which has provoked another person to behave in an unpleasant way.

The other two antecedent strategy types are cognitive, and comprise the steering of attention and the manner of appraising the situation. Steering of attention concerns the management of information absorption, and consists of directing attention away from or to specific parts of the situation and/or associated thoughts and/or experiences. Regulation of appraisal may consist of decisions to interpret a situation in a specific way (for instance as a challenge rather than a problem). It may also consist of a reconsideration of a situation in order to provoke positive- rather than negative emotions.

Table 8.3 Overview of main factors in emotion regulation

Situation–Attention–Appraisal	Emotional reaction tendencies	Emotional response
	↓	↓
Antecedent regulations	Behavior Experience Physiological Responses	Reaction-based regulations

Based on Gross (1998) and Gross & Thompson (2007)

Reaction-based regulation focus are those that are directly concerned with increasing, decreasing or maintain emotional tension. «Repression» in this context, together with «suppression», is considered as an emotion regulation strategy. Other examples may be to ignore emotions, distract oneself by thinking about something else and/or engage in social (talk with somebody), cognitive (read, listen to music, look at a video) or physical (carpentry, painting, or exercise) distraction activities. The examples may show that situation focused and reaction-based strategies may blend with each other, which come naturally because Table 8.3 shows moments of a process rather than clearly differentiated phenomena.

Gross and co-workers' studies have been directed at exploring the consequences and variations of two regulation strategies: «Reappraisal», which is an antecedent-based cognitive strategy, and «suppression» which is a reaction-based strategy. A central study consisted of having 40 students each in one of three groups attend to two short emotion arousing films of treatment of bruins and amputation of an arm. The measures included ratings to indicate emotional experience, measurement of finger temperature and GSR to indicate physiological reactions, and measures of emotional expression and behavior base scoring of recording of behavior during the films. Experimental manipulations were made in terms of instructions to the groups. Students in one group were «naive» and were simply told to look at the films, a second group was a «reappraisal group» where participants were told to be neutral and focus on the technical parts of the treatments on the film, and a third group was a «suppression group» where participants were told to suppress their emotional reactions so that they could not be observed by anybody which might watch them (Gross, 1998).

The results showed that students in both strategy-groups reduced their behavior as compared to students in the naive group, that the reappraisal group participants rated reduced experience of emotions, and that the suppression group participants had fewer physiological reactions than the others. These differences have since been repeated with specific emotions such as happiness and sadness. It has also been shown that suppression has negative consequences for the interaction with others, and that both strategies are used to different degree by different persons. Results from this research also suggested that reappraisal is associated with a more healthy lifestyle and better health than suppression (Gross, 1998; Gross & John, 2003; John & Gross, 2004).

Gross and co-workers have convincingly shown that an intensive mapping of individual strategies is necessary to gain full insight into emotion regulation. The limitation of the research is that it only comprises two strategies and has failed to provide a reason for the focus on reappraisal and suppression rather than other strategies. It would for instance be important to know if these two strategies are especially common, or if they have especially large or central consequences. There may be some further insight to be gained from an approach to a description of the distribution of emotion regulation strategies.

8.5 Parkinson and Totterdell's Map of Emotion Regulation Strategies

Koole (2009) has proposed an overview over emotion regulation types by differentiating between three different targets and functions. The proposal comprises no information about which strategies or types that are actually used. Answers to this question are more likely to follow a track indicated by Parkinson and Totterdell (1999), who designed the most comprehensive study which has been conducted pertaining to mapping persons' emotion regulation strategies. The mapping was based on descriptions from a group of students in response to questionnaires of people's manner of improving their negative emotion. Another group of participants was interviewed directly, and yet another group completed a diary of how they had actually regulated their emotions during a day. The study comprised a total of 150 participants. The descriptions were supplied by responses from 116 students who were asked to describe what they did to cheer up themselves when they did not feel very well.

The first rough classification of responses resulted in a sample of 304 emotion regulation strategies. The resulting selection when strategies with the same meaning were included in the same category was a sample of 162 strategies. Statistical analyses in order to identify the underlying strategies led to the final classification of 13 types which are shown in Table 8.4 (see page 61).

Table 8.4 shows two main types of strategies, cognitive and behavioral, which were either used as a diversion from- or as an engagement to an emotional situation. All these strategies pertain to the reaction-based type in Gross' model. Table 8.4 shows, furthermore, that Gross' reappraisal strategy, which was conceived as antecedent-based, is classified as a reaction-based cognitive engagement strategy by Parkinson and Totterdell, and that Gross' cognitive strategy probably pertain to the cognitive disengagement strategy in Table 8.4. Table 8.4 also may seem to assimilate the avoidant coping strategy as disengagement regulation, and the problem- and emotion-focused coping strategies as, respectively, cognitive and behavioral engagement strategies in Fig. 35 (see Sect. 7.4).

The significance of Parkinson and Totterdell' results may be somewhat unclear. One reason for this is that the participants mainly responded in relation to memories rather than direct experiences. This may raise some questions, but it is not a definitive problem. Research has shown that there is good agreement between the description of the actual experience of emotions and reports based on the memory for the experience (Feldman Barrett, 2006). Another reason for unclearness about the significance of the results is that the strategies in Table 8.4 are based on a limited sample of emotions.

Table 8.4 Parkinson and Totterdell's (1999, p. 300) classification of emotion regulation strategies

	Cognitive	Behavioural
DIVERSION		
Disengagement	Avoid thinking about the problem	Avoid problematic situation
Distraction		
Seek pleasure or relaxation	Think about something pleasant Think about relaxing thoughts	Do something pleasant Do something relaxing
Reallocate resources	Think about something that occupies attention	Perform a demanding activity
ENGAGEMENT		
	Reappraise (usually affect-directed)	Vent feelings (usually affect-directed Seek help or comfort from others)
	Think about how to solve problem (usually situation-directed)	Take action to solve problem (usually situation-directed)

The participants were only questioned about their manners of reducing emotional tension, and only in relation to negative emotions. The fact that the sample only consisted of 266 persons from the same cultural area (England and USA) is also not very convincing as a background for a classification of all relevant emotion regulation strategies.

8.6 Supplementary Studies and Remaining Problems

The results from Parkinson and Totterdell's study showed a distribution of regulation strategies, but did not comprise and indication of the most preferred or effective strategies. Supplementary studies in this context was conducted by Vikan, Dias, & Nordvik (2009) and Vikan, Rugseth, & Hassel (2010), who administered questionnaires to 401 Brazilian and 418 Norwegian students as well as 200 patients from outpatient clinics about their use and perceived efficiency of 14 strategies to stop being angry, sad, or anxious. The strategies represented the main types in Table 8.4. The results showed that the 1018 participants agreed about five of the 14 strategies as the ones they preferred. Top strategies were: «Say something to oneself», «Think of doing something else or forget the emotion», and «Begin to work with something». The most frequently selected strategies were also those that were rated as most effective. All participants selected more than one strategy for each emotion, the mean selection was 6 strategies.

The results also showed some cultural differences. "Go for a walk", and «Acting out the emotion» was, for instance, more often selected by Norwegian than by Brazilian students, whereas «Relaxation» and «Entertainment» was more often used by the Brazilians. The study showed in addition clinical differences and differences related to emotion type. «Avoid others» was, for instance proposed much more often by patients than by non-patients, and «Go for a walk» was more often proposed as a strategy to regulate anger and sadness than to regulate fear.

The participants' efficiency ratings may not be reliable indicators of strategy efficiency. This should at least be supplied by comparisons of the effect of different strategies such as in Gross' (1998) study. An overview of results from 190 studies of this type has indicated that the most efficient regulation strategies are reappraisal, objectivation of one's relation to the emotion arousing stimulus or event, and active distraction (Webb, Miles, & Sheeran, 2012). The overview showed that all studies have comprised cognitive strategies, and that the most frequent targets of regulation has been negative emotions generally, and anger, sadness, and fear specifically. Disgust and happiness have also appeared in a few studies.

It should be noted in closing this presentation that the variation in strategies may be much larger than the ones indicated in Sects. 8.4 and 8.5. There is, for instance, a lack of tests for regulation strategies of a majority of the emotions which are described in Chap. 3. Variations in emotion regulation associated with cultural variation (see Chap. 9) and mental health problems (Kring & Werner, 2004) may also be much larger than what is indicated in Gross' model and Parkinson and Totterdell's results. A comprehensive list of strategies should also comprise newborn's tension reduction reflexes and all types of regulation noted in Tables 8.1 and 8.2 (see also Bargh & Williams, 2007). It may seem that there is a need for many additional studies before emotion regulation can be more than a useful concept for how emotional responses may be influenced.

8.7 Practical Relevance

Emotion regulation is a concept which is easily adapted for practical use. Challenges of emotion regulation are very frequent for all who raise children or work with children in a professional capacity. Ways and strategies of emotion regulation is, furthermore, a main task in psychotherapy, in coaching and in discussions and development of the co-operative climate at work. A first and central point is to be conscious of one's regulation strategies, the emotion work which is involved, and the personal and social consequences associated with each strategy. This makes possible an awareness of how strategies may be modified in order to be in accordance with one's goals in life. It may be especially useful to do a mapping both of "feeling rules" and regulation strategies by partners in relationships and participants in groups (especially from different cultures) as prevention of misunderstandings and conflicts.

8.8 Summary

A short to-the-point definition of emotion regulation is: «... the processes involved in modifying emotional reactions». Emotion regulation is, unlike coping, easily related to individual emotions and target the emotion itself rather than a stressful situation.

Emotion regulation is first shown in infants in terms of reflexive reactions to reduce tension, such as head-turning and disengagement of attention. The infant learn new manners of regulation emotions from about three months of age in interaction with their CP. This can result in general manners of handling emotions as the infants' attachment is stabilized in the sixth or seventh month. The child starts to use cognitive regulation and be influenced by moral norms in its third year, and has established the basis of an internalized, independent basis of regulation in the fourth to fifth year.

Emotion regulation at birth and in the first year is motivated by the need to maintain an inner, organismic balance (homeostasis). Inner motivation for regulation in adolescents and adults may be to obtain an optimal intensity level and to keeping the person well organized. An additional, social motivation in terms of norms is added in the course of development. The norms are, according to Hochschild (1979) , "feeling rules" which prescribe when, where, and to what extent individual emotions should be experienced and expressed. The effort to regulate emotions to comply with norms has been denoted as "emotion work", and described as surface and deep acting.

Two main approaches have been made in order to classify emotion regulation strategies. Gross has made a distinction between four types of antecedent- and one type reaction-based regulation strategies in relation to a theoretical sequence of emotional causation, and Parkinson and Totterdell have identified 13 types distributed into cognitive and behavioral diversion and engagement strategies.

Studies have indicated that there may be cultural similarities in the use of regulation strategies, but that there are also indications of variation related to cultural values and to emotion type.

Reflection Questions

1. What are your regulation strategies for decrease your anger and fear, and what strategies do you use to be happy? How would you rate your strategies in terms of effectivity and health?
2. Some people seem to get stuck in very unhealthy emotion regulation strategies that provide powerful double gain by producing positive- and avoiding negative emotions at the same time. One example may be alcoholic intoxication (alcoholism), another may be drug dependency. Do you know other examples, and are there also healthy double-gain strategies?

Research/Exercise Examples

1. Antecedent regulation refers to what people do to avoid and seek out situations to, respectively avoid negative emotions and experience positive ones. You and your fellow students may get an example of the scope and importance of emotional regulation by trying to map how you plan and arrange your behavior during a normal day to avoid negative and obtain positive emotions.
2. Are rules for the expression of the emotions of anger, fear, and sadness mostly related to individual experiences, peer-group interaction or socialization in families? This is a question about central influences on emotional behavior, and you can get some cues for a discussion from descriptions of your own and each of your parents' emotion rules and from those of the others in your student group as well as their parents. Descriptions should also be checked for differences in gender and parents' education.

Further Reading

Gross, J. J. (Ed.). (2007). *Handbook of emotion regulation*. New York: The Guilford Press.

Vikan, A., Dias, M., & Nordvik, H. (2009). Perceived efficiency and use of strategies for emotion regulation. *Psychological Reports, 104,* 455–467.

Webb, T. L., Miles, E., & Sheeran, P. (2012). Dealing with feeling: A meta-analysis of the effectiveness of strategies derived from the process model of emotion regulation. *Psychological Bulletin, 138,* 775–808.

Emotion and Culture

9

Teil I

Emotions unite us and separate us. Descriptions in Sects. 2.6 and 5.1.3 show, respectively, that facial expressions of six basic emotions are recognized by people all over the world, and that we speak the same emotional language when we are about one year old. We have also referred to examples that persons may unconsciously imitate and infect each other's emotions. This chapter is, in contrast to these examples, introduced by very different emotional behaviors in three non-Western cultural environments. This will be supported by several other examples that emotions are dependent on, or relative to cultural factors, an are examples of a relativistic viewpoint was for many years the dominant one and supported by Klineberg's (1954) influential textbook. Ekman (Ekman, Friesen, & Ellsworth, 1972) and Izard (1971) were, therefore, met with mistrust and strong criticism when they argued that emotions are universal and supported this with results from the cross-cultural studies of agreement on photos of facial expressions which cited in Sect. 2.6. The universality position and its opposition are shown in more detail in, respectively, Izard's and Russell/Feldman Barret's modern theories in Chap. 11. This chapter is continued with additional examples of universality and a description of viewpoints and studies related to emotions in individualistic and collectivistic cultures. The final part of the chapter is a short presentation of emotional gender cultures.

9.1 Emotions in Three Cultures

Many descriptions of ancient societies, for instance the Spartans and the Vikings, and of non-technological tribes, for instance 39 tribes in Papua New Guinea (Diamond, 2012), depict people as preoccupied with aggressive emotions. Adults are described as constantly preparing either for defending themselves or for making warfare or going on robbery, their daily life is described as showing frequent acts of aggression and they are held to raise their children to be quarrelsome and aggressively competitive.

There is a marked contrast between the aggressive cultures and the Utku-eskimos, who show practically no anger at all. The Utkus conceive of anger as a loss of control which may lead to all kinds of negative events, inclusive murder. Their behavior is characterized by tolerance and quietness, and they are cautious in order to avoid provocations of anger in their social interactions. They were also consistently tolerant towards the anthropologist Briggs (1970), who lived with them for about a year. This ended in the spring, when the Utkus were visited by a group of tourists. The tourists borrowed some of the Utku's kayaks without asking, and did some harm to them because of their lack of experience. Briggs got angry, scolded the tourists for lacking respect for the Utku culture, and demanded that they should apologize and compensate the Utkus for the damage. The Utkus overheard Briggs' diatribe and asked her to leave their community because they could not trust a person who expressed anger openly in relation to other persons.

Anger is neither a wanted nor a forbidden emotion on Bali, Indonesia. But anger is not welcome. It should, in all instances, be replaced by happiness, which is not a theme in the other two cultures. Happiness should according to Balinese culture be the main element in all social interaction. It is a strong Balinese norm that persons should keep their front and show a smile. It is an expectation, a demand, and almost a command that persons should be happy and forget what occurred if some negative event has happened. Joking and telling humorous stories are frequently employed to amuse and to suppress negative emotions (Wikan, 1990).

These three examples leave little doubt that emotional behavior, expression or regulation can be very different in different cultures. The emotions may even seem to define the different cultural patterns. This suggests a culture-relativistic interpretation of emotions, i.e. that emotions are dependent on, or relative to cultural characteristics. A relativistic viewpoint may seem as natural as a universalistic viewpoint that emotions are independent of culture. The relativistic viewpoint may even seem more obvious because cultures vary in their organization, comprise different interpretations of the world and of human existence and includes different values and norms for behavior. The aggressive cultures, the Utkus', and the Balinese's differences in world views as suggested by differences in emotion regulations may be parallel to the differences in emotional reactions related to different instructions in Lazarus and Alfert's (1964) study (see Sect. 6.1.1).

A. Vikan, *A Fast Road to the Study of Emotions*,
DOI 10.1007/978-3-319-52313-2_9

9.2 Relativism

Support for a relativistic viewpoint is most clearly provided by studies of historical descriptions of emotions and variations of emotion terms in different languages, and by results from studies of emotion regulation and emotional behavior.

Historical descriptions show variation especially in terms of the importance of control of emotions. Control is generally represented as suppression of anger and/or of expressions of "weakness" (sadness, shame, guilt and compassion). Spartan and Roman cultures are well known examples of such control. A more recent example is Elias' (2000) description of the low degree of emotional control in European culture in the late middle age period which was increased as part of a civilizing process in the following centuries. Another example is Stearns and Stearns (1986) description of three stages of increased control of aggression in the U.S.A. from the eighteenth century to about 1970 (see also Matt, 2011).

Other historical indications of relativism are descriptions of «historical» types of emotions. An example is "acedia", which was a depressive state characterized by an experience of lack of meaning which was much discussed in literature in the Middle Ages (Harre and Finlay-Jones, 1986).

Variations in linguistic expressions of emotions are very evident in the number of emotion words. There are, for example, about 400 words for emotions in the English language, about 750 in Chinese, 230 in Malay, and only 8 in the Chewong-language in Malay (Heelas, 1986). The words for emotions also do not correspond to each other. The English language has several words for varieties of an emotion which is covered by only one word in other languages. English may, furthermore, have one word each for two different emotions, such as "sad" and "angry", which is referred to by one and the same word in an African languages (Leff, 1973). One description of linguistic variations is that cultures may be hypercognitive (have many words) or hypocognitive (have only a few words) in referring to specific emotions, as, for instance, Tahitian references to, respectively, anger and sadness (Levy, 1984).

Words and expressions for emotions in different languages may, furthermore, be partly overlapping. Other languages may refer to emotions like in the English language, but both English and a given another language may have words for emotions that do not exist in the other. The word "emotion" is adapted from English common language and lacks an exact parallel in other languages such as French, German, and Russian. The variation in words also pertains to basic emotions. Russell (1991) showed in an overview that words for happiness, surprise, fear, sadness, and disgust are all lacking in one or more languages and that the word for anger is overlapping for sadness or grief in African languages and languages in the Pacific.

The convincing evidence for linguistic variation has not, except in Russell and Feldman Barrett's theory (see Sect. 11.4.2), been a decisive argument in discussions about emotions. The main reason for this is that experience and consciousness are not identical to language. One example is that children show a variation of emotions long before they know any words for these emotions. Another example is Levy's (1973) note that the inhabitants in Tahiti lack a word for sadness, but they show very clear signs of sadness and grief when they have lost a person in their family. It has been argued that variations in linguistic expressions may be anchored in the same (universal) emotional experience because word may refer to different facets of an emotional process (in terms of causes, appraisals, expressions, and behavior) in different cultures (Mesquita & Frijda, 1992).

It can be added that emotions are experienced by language users and not by languages. Enumeration of words in a given language do not necessarily show how these words are used, and nothing at all about how the language user can refer to her/his emotional experiences by other words than those which refer directly to emotions.

Variations in emotion regulation. The description in Sect. 9.1 of large differences between cultures may be seen as examples of differences in emotion regulation. There are many examples of descriptions of culture-related emotion regulation in anthropological literature. The "classical" example is Margaret Mead's (1935) report from three tribes in New Guinea. The large differences between the aggressive, hostile Mungudumor- and the passive and peaceful Arapesh tribes described by Mead show similar differences to that between the aggressive- and Utku societies. Both examples suggest a dimension of emotion regulation from societies with relatively openly expressed aggression (e.g. U.S.A) to societies where aggression is suppressed and is attributed a relatively low value (e.g. Japan) which is often displayed in cross-cultural comparisons. Other examples of suppressed emotions are the Hare-indians in Canada, who suppress expressions of jealousy, happiness, and anger, «prohibitions» against romantic emotions in Beduin cultures, and suppression of all forms of emotional expressions in the Chewong people in Malaya (Mesquita and Frijda, 1992).

Variations in behavior. "Behavior" in this context comprises other than facial expressions of emotions, such as the voice, gesticulation, and the orientation and movements of the body. Results from studies have shown similarities in use of voice and physiological signals of different emotions (see Sect. 4.2) (Scherer, Wallbott, & Summerfield, 1986), but variations are generally much more salient. This is because cultural cognitive patterns and values are most visibly expressed in behavior in comparable social situations. The emotions in weddings and funerals are, for instance expressed differently in ritualized behavior and symbolic colors by different cultures. Differences in cultural patterns are the reason that behavior of people in one culture may be considered as «incomprehensible» or «meaningless» by people from another. Niedenthal, Krauth-Gruber, and Ric (2006) mentioned as an example that a dead body arouses disgust in all known cultures except in Navajo-indians, who experience intense fear because they think that dead bodies are invaded by dangerous spirits.

Other cultural variations. Some researchers have interpreted cultural variations as support for an emotional relativism which means that emotions are specific to the culture in which they appear. Happiness, anger, and fear as experienced by people in one culture is, thus, conceived as different from the happiness, anger, and fear which is experienced by people in another culture. A main support or this is that persons in some cultures seem to harbor emotions which are unknown to persons in other cultures. An example is Lutz' (1988) description of the emotion "metagu" in people at the Ifaluk islands in the Pacific ocean. "Metagu" refers to a mild anxious caring for others which has not been observed (or described) in persons in other cultures. Lutz also described other examples of unknown or unusual emotions, and chose the title "unnatural emotions" for the book he wrote after his stay at the island.

9.3 Universality

Support for universality are most frequently shown in cross-cultural studies of recognition of facial expressions, appraisals of links between causes and emotions, and experiences of physiological signals.

Recognition of facial expressions. Design and results from the most comprehensive studies were cited in Sect. 2.5. The account here is therefore limited to a presentation of Ekman and co-workers' study that included participation from members of the Fore tribe in New Guinea (Ekman, 1973). The tribe had only had minimal contact with other tribes or peoples, and the members could, consequently, not have learnt facial expressions from others in more dominant cultures. Testing for recognition of facial expressions was conducted in two parts. The first part consisted of reading the same stories comprising emotions to Fore tribe members and U.S students and ask them to select one of three pictures of facial expression to show the emotion in the story. The results were that adult members of the Fore tribe and U.S students selected about the same pictures.

The second part of the study consisted of instructing tribe members to show their facial expression in response to typical events. The events which were read to the tribe members were:

(a) *Your friend has come and you are happy*
(b) *Your child has died*
(c) *You are angry and about to fight*
(d) *You see a dead pig which has been lying there for a long time*

The Fore facial expressions related to each of these events were photographed and shown to U.S. students who were asked to name the emotion shown on the photograph. The results were that the students generally selected emotion words that corresponded to the facial expression represented by the tribespeople. The results of both parts support an interpretation that facial expressions are universal.

It can be noted that these results were less dependent on emotion words than the study cited at length in Sect. 2.5, and therefore less subject to Russell's (1991, 1994) criticism. It can also be reminded that the real agreement on emotional expressions between the very different cultures in the New Guinea study may be higher than is shown by testing for identification of emotions in photographs. The reason is that photographs lack many of the cues which are ordinarily associated with facial expressions, such as context (situation) and the intensity and timing of the emotional response.

Appraisals of links between causes and emotions. Methodological problems pertaining to use of words and photographs can, to some extent, be counteracted by testing whether emotions are systematically and cross-culturally linked to causal situations. Results from this approach has supported face recognition results by showing a high degree of agreement among persons from different cultures about which type of situations are linked as causes and/or arousing events of anger, disgust, fear, sadness, happiness, surprise, and jealousy. The exception is comparatively low agreements in comparisons which include persons from parts of the world were the context consists of unique environments such as the arctic and desert environments. The most frequent causes, especially for anger, sadness, and happiness, are stimuli or events related to encounters with other persons (Scherer et al., 1986).

Studies within this approach have also comprised tests for the degree to which situations are appraised as pleasant, surprising or related to a goal. High agreement in appraisals have been shown in results from comparisons of persons from the U.S. and Japan and in Wallbott and Scherer's (1988) study with participants from 27 countries from different continents. Thus, the conclusion seems to be that there are generally high cross-cultural similarities about the differential relations between situations and emotions. But a premise is that the objective situation is interpreted more or less in the same way. This is not always the case. A study with children from China and the U.S. showed, for example, that the Chinese showed a tendency of interpreting sadness in situations where the Americans interpreted aggression (Borke & Su, 1972).

Emotional changes in the body. It can be assumed that the physiological function of the body leads to parallel changes associated with emotions all over the world. This is supported by experiences related to anger, happiness, fear, and sadness in persons from Europe and the U.S.A. (Scherer et al., 1986). The similarities comprised changes related to signs for shame, disgust, and guilt which are shown in Table 4.3 and which was based on reports from persons from 27 countries (Wallbott & Scherer, 1988). Similar results have been reported by Breugelmans et al. (2005).

9.4 What Do Cultural Differences Show? Individualism and Collectivism

Universality has, as was referred to in Sect. 2.5 been explained since Darwin's times as based on inherited circuits in the brain. This is a biological interpretation of emotions which are detailed in Chap. 11. Relativism has been explained by reference to culture. Culture comprises persons' patterns of norms, attitudes, values, world-views, social organization, and behavior, and represents a social interpretation of emotions. The references to culture in Sects. 9.1 and 9.2 only show that culture is a factor or a variable which results in different emotional reactions. The differences in responses do not in themselves

Table 9.1 Key words for characteristics of collectivistic and individualistic cultures

	Collectivism	*Individualism*
Fokus	Relation to in-group	The person her-/himself
Family	Parents, siblings, grandparents aunts, uncles, cousins, etc.	Nuclear family (mother, father, siblings)
Upbringing	Compliance, conformity	Independence
Orientation of self	Dependency	Self reliance
General orientation	Norms, obligation, others' expectations	Own priorities, needs, wants and plans
Value and emotion	Honor and shame	Self-realization and guilt

show how emotions are part of a cultural expression. They do not, for example, show how emotions are parts of a pattern of regulation related to norms and values, or how they serve to articulate individuals and their selves in community with others (Lutz & White, 1986).

An attempt to relate emotions to a more extensive concept of culture is represented by Markus and Kitayama's (1994) discussion of the positive valuation of anger in the U.S. as compared to the negative valuation of the emotion in Japan. The authors held that valuation is related to the U.S. concept of the individual as independent from other's and as responsible only for her/himself as compared to the Japanese concept of the individual as reciprocally dependent on and responsible for her/his group. This, they argued, leads to a perception of anger as an important tool to obtain an individual's goals in the U.S and as a disturbance to group interactions in Japan. This difference is characteristic of, respectively, individualistic and collectivistic cultures, which are the cultural patterns which have most often been linked to differences in emotional experiences, expressions, and behavior.

Individualism and collectivism pertain, very simplified, to the relation between the individual and her/his closest group (in-group). Individualism is mainly characteristic of cultures in Western Europe and in North America, and implies that individuals experience themselves as independent of their groups and with responsibility mainly or only towards themselves. Persons are focused on self-expression and personal achievement, which leads to pride in success and anger in failure. These emotions empathize the individual at the expense of the group, and has been called "disengaging emotions" (Niedenthal et al., 2006).

Collectivism is characteristic of cultures in Eastern Asia, Africa, Southern Europe and South America, and implies that individuals experience themselves as part of their closest group, which is ordinarily the family, and with responsibility first and foremost to this group. Persons are focused on reciprocal identity and attachment with the group. This leads to frequent positive emotions related to friendship and respect, and to shame and guilt when something happens that breaks the reciprocal harmony. These emotions have, accordingly, been called "engaging emotions" by Niedenthal et al. (2006). An overview of differences between individualistic and collectivistic emotions is shown in Table 9.1 (top of page).

Results from studies have shown that individualism is associated with a tendency to use force and aggression and to be inconsiderate and ruthless. This is also indicated by results from studies where persons in individualistic cultures also have been reported to express their emotions intensely, accept aggressive emotions, give high intensity accept ratings of disengagement emotions and communicate a relatively wide variety of emotions (Earley & Gibson, 1998; Matsumoto et al., 2008). Results from studies of persons in collectivistic cultures have shown that they tend to a high valuation of positive- and to suppress negative emotions, and to show high acceptance ratings of engagement emotions (Hammer & Gudykunst, 1986; Porter & Samovar, 1998). Note that these characteristics correspond to the Utku and Balinese collectivistic cultures in Sect. 9.1, but not for the valuation of anger in the likewise collectivistic aggressive cultures.

9.5 Gender Differences

Women and men may seem as pertaining to two different emotional cultures. Results from several studies suggest that women experience more intense, lasting, and frequent emotions than men, that they notice emotions in themselves and others better than men, and that women have better memory for emotions and expresses their emotions more strongly and with more marked facial expressions (Fischer, 1993, Niedenthal et al., 2006). Some of this may be due to biological differences, such as boys' higher level of activity and greater difficulty of being calmed than girls, who initiates contact with others more frequently and react stronger to distress in others Brody, 2000).

Interpretations of these differences have mainly been related to social factors, e.g. social roles and differences in upbringing, but have been limited by the fact that practically all studies have been conducted within a Western European-North American cultural context. There has therefore been no guarantee that differences are also shown outside of this restricted cultural space. This may have been remedied by analyzes on a database which comprise ratings of intensity, duration and expression of seven different emotions from 2917 participants in 37 countries (Fischer & Manstead, 2000). The general result was that gender differences shown in individualistic cultures were not as large but were also shown in collectivistic cultures. This may, according to the authors, mean that gender differences have a biological basis which may vary with the masculinity of cultural values, women's part-taking in a society's working life and economy, and the distribution of work in family life.

9.6 Culture or Biology?

Discussions whether emotions are biologically or culturally founded have been intense up to the present. The extreme viewpoint on the biological side, which we have referred to several times, is that emotions are inherited, hardwired in the brain, are more or less identical with the facial expression and lasts less than a minute (e.g. Ekman, 1972). The extreme viewpoint on the cultural side is that emotions are what are referred to by the words which are used in talk about emotions (e.g. Harre, 1986). This means, in relation to the definition of emotions in 1. 1., that experiential component of emotions tend to be ignored by the extreme biological viewpoint and to be the only type of components which are considered by the extreme cultural viewpoint.

The difference in viewpoints may be framed in the traditional genotype-phenotype distinction, where genotype represents a hardwired, hereditary biological influence, and phenotype refers to culturally variable experiential and behavioral components.

The presentation in the present chapter suggests that this represents factors which are jointly influencing the coordination of the three components which were defined as emotions in the present book (Sect. 1.3). The genotype biological view is historically dominating, but there is probably little disagreement today that culture, in terms of learning, modifies the phenotype of a handful of "basic emotions" (Sect. 1.9) in the first year of the child's life (see Sect. 5.1). There may be a little more disagreement about an argument that emotions which are primarily social and presuppose self-consciousness (see Sect. 5.2) cannot *not* be anchored in the CNS i.e., show some biological influence. The remaining disagreement, therefore, should not be whether emotions show influence from one or the other set of factors, but in what way and to what extent each individual emotion is influenced by both biological and cultural factors.

The suggestion from Sect. 1.9 and Chap. 5 is that this type of discussion should be related to a differentiation between basic and social emotions and to a development of emotions from prototypical to ordinary and include the self-conscious emotions. Biological factors may, for instance, be conceived as decisive for the prototypical basic emotions and as a necessary basis for the first ordinary emotions, whereas cultural factors may be conceived as contributing to the development of ordinary emotions and as dominant for the development of self-conscious emotions. An overview of indications of relativistic and universal aspects of emotions from the present chapter as well as from the subsequent Chap. 11 is shown in Table 9.2.

9.7 Practical Relevance

This chapter comprises central practical aims in relation to contact, communication, and cooperation across cultural borders. Results from the studies which have been cited may indicate that one may fail both easily and definitively. Persons from different cultures amuse themselves by roughly the same entertainment, fear the same dangers, and get sad for corresponding events. But the responses are at the same time embedded in different cultures and related to different values. The lack of insight into this and the failure to develop practices to show each other how we differ in our links to the same reality may be costly indeed. The examples are that our amusement also may be others' offence, and that the reactions that follow may be increased many times by individual emotional reactions which infect large groups and results in loss of life and large material destruction.

The cultural encounters with their complexities of universal reactions and culturally dependent appraisals are happening in partnerships and families, in kindergartens, schools, the social and health support institutions and the places of work. And they happen to an increased degree in trade and industrial enterprises which are becoming dependent on diversification and global cooperation. The possibilities to succeed on these different levels depends on an understanding of how our emotions and that of others are the same and different because of our cultural differences.

9.8 Summary

Emotions may be affected mainly by biological factors and be universal, or by cultural factors and be relativistic. Variations in historical descriptions of emotions and in words for emotions

Table 9.2 Overview of indications of relativistic and universal aspects of emotion

Relativistic indications	*Universal indications*
Different emotions shown at different historical phases	Cross-cultural agreement on relation of facial expressions and emotion names
Cultural variation in motion words	Cross-cultural agreement on causes of emotions
Cultural variation in regulation of emotions	Cross-cultural agreement on physiological signals
Variation in behavioral expression of emotions	General indications of emotional arousal (Chap. 11)
Variation in meaning with cultural patterns	Variation with arousal in emotion type (Chap. 11)

in different languages can suggest that emotions are formed by cultural factors. Cultural relativism is also indicated by observations that emotions are regulated in different ways and are expressed by very different behaviors in different cultures around the world. A further indication of relativism is that there seems to be specific types of emotions in isolated societies.

Universal qualities of emotions are, on the other hand, suggested by results from studies which show that persons from isolated societies both display facial expressions of emotions and recognize emotional facial expressions which are, respectively, recognized by and in accordance with persons in modern societies. Universality is also suggested by agreement among persons from different cultures about which causes are related to specific emotions such as fear, anger, and happiness, and in experiences of physiological signals of different emotions.

Cultural variation has been related to concepts of individualistic and collectivistic cultures. Emotions in individualistic cultures, where focus is on the individual's independence and responsibilities toward her/himself, are expressed in greater variation and intensity than emotions in collectivistic cultures, where the focus is on the individual's dependency on and responsibilities towards her/his closest groups. Individualistic persons show, furthermore, high valuing of disengagement emotions like anger and pride, in contrast to collectivistic persons' high valuing of engagement emotions like happiness, shame, and guilt.

Studies in a variation of cultures seem to support conclusions that women's experiences are more frequent, intense, and lasting, and are expressed more clearly than men's emotional experiences. This difference seems to be larger in individualistic than in collectivistic cultures.

Modern views recognize that emotions are affected both by biological and cultural factors, and may affect different types of emotions, i.e. basic and social emotions, in different ways. Basic emotions seem to be affected mainly by biological- and social emotions mainly by cultural factors.

Reflection Questions

1. Imagine yourself suddenly transformed to as culture which is very different from your own and whose language you do not know e.g. such as the Fore in New Guinea.
   How would you try to learn emotional reactions and rules? What types of error would you be most likely to make?
2. Emotions are related to values, and values are building blocks of cultures. Emotional expressions of cultural conflict, or cultural conflicts that seem totally deadlocked often refer to actual or perceived violation of cultural values. Are there examples in the media of conflicts between groups, countries and/or religious communities who comprise this type of reactions? Do you also know conflicts which have been diminished or practically eliminated by reciprocal emotional respect?

Research/Exercise Examples

1. A straightforward test of cultural variation would be to interview samples of persons from different cultures about causes and rules of expression of emotions. The significance of results would be increased if causes were focused on relevant events (you are wanted or not wanted by someone, you win or lose the competition with someone, you fail or succeed at some matter, you want something from someone, someone betrays you, you steal something from someone or have something stolen from you, your parents approve or disapprove of you in some way…).
   What cultures would you include in such a study, and why? It may be difficult to find cultural representatives in your surroundings, but could the study be conducted on the net? How?
2. Culture differences may also be shown as historical differences. You can test this by checking on the emotional culture in your country/culture in the most ancient novels available at the general library in your town. Historians or folklorists might tell you whether there are other literature, for instance moral advice, which also could show the main concepts of emotions and emotional expression at the time.

Further Reading

Kitayama, S., & Markus, H. R. (Eds.). (1994). *Emotion and culture: Empirical studies of mutual influence*. Washington, D. C.: American Psychological Association.

Mesquita, B. (2001). Emotions in collectivist and individualist contexts. *Journal of Personality and Social Psychology, 80*, 68–74.

Wallbott, H. G., & Scherer, K. R. (1986). How universal and specific is emotional experience? Evidence from 27 countries on five continents. *Social Science Information, 25*, 763–795.

Emotions in the Workplace 10

The major part of people's emotional life takes place in social contexts, such as families, schools, churches, workplaces, restaurants, sports arenas, and cinemas. These may at times be set up to release specific emotions, such as happiness (the family during Christmas), interest (the school) or fear, anger, and/or happiness (cinemas), and influence or be influenced differently by the arousal, regulation and expression of emotions.

There is very little information on this emotional ecology, and it is not within the scope of the present book. This chapter comprises a survey of emotions in the workplace because this has been the main source for the salient concepts of emotion work and emotional intelligence. The chapter is also included because of the economic significance of emotions in contributing to the productivity and creativity of the workforce in organizations which are the nave of society's economic life. Thus, emotions should be an economic concern in addition to being a concern of individual behavior, social interaction, mental and physical health, and cultural transactions.

The chapter begins with a survey of the general recognition of emotional processes in the workplace, continues with a presentation of the concept of emotions work, and is closed with a discussion of emotional intelligence.

10.1 Emotions in the Workplace

Several authors have pointed out that although emotions are fundamental and always present in the workplace, their role in everyday activity have been pejoratively considered and they have been practically ignored by systematic analyses (e.g. Ashforth & Humprey, 1995; Matthews, Zeidner, & Roberts, 2002). A reason for this neglect is an illusion that organizations are fully rational, that emotions scarcely exist at the workplace and that they certainly do not influence on work. The illusion was, according to Ashforth and Humphrey (1995), fostered by an administrative paradigm of rationality and maintained by four mechanisms to regulate emotions which are shown in Table 10.1(see page 70).

The illusion of rationality is paradoxical because the functioning of an organization is dependent on powerful drivers such as interest and happiness related to success, and anger, shame, and fear related to failure. The attachment of emotions to the organization's duties and goals decide the degree to which attention and effort is directed at them (George & Brief, 1996). And triggers at the workplace for all emotions in Chap. 3 are easily envisaged. Happiness is, for instance, triggered by meaningful challenges and success, anger by being treated unjustly, betrayed, and blocked, fear by threats and/or accusations, sadness by failures, loss, and refusals, shame by inadequate performances, pride by personal and organizational success, and envy by others' competences, qualities and position.

There have been attempts to classify work-related emotions (Hochschild, 2003; Pekrun & Frese, 1992) although emotions at the workplace are not different from emotions elsewhere. They influence and are influenced in the same ways as those which have been described in the other parts of this book. This means, for instance, that the large part of employees whose duties are performed directly in contact with others are constantly exposed to others' faces (see Sect. 2.6) and are, consequently, infected subcortically by others' emotions (see Sect. 4.6) which triggers reactions in muscles and/or intestines (see Sects. 4.2 and 12.2), resonates on the self (see Sect. 4.4), influences employees' perception of the other and the interaction (see Sect. 4.1) and their thinking about the problems at hand (Sect. 6.2), and are felt as drives toward certain behaviors (see Sect. 1.5) and must be regulated (see Sect. 8.3) according to social rules. The emotion may, furthermore, result in a biased memory of the interaction (see Sect. 6.2) and a need to talk to someone (see Sect. 4.7) about the client and the interaction.

There is little knowledge about how these processes are related to the workplace. The significance of emotions is indicated by studies which have shown that stress and satisfaction at the workplace may influence the productivity of the organization and the physical and mental health of employees (see Sect. 7.4). But stress and satisfaction are general concepts that represent information neither on specific emotions nor on specific organizational outcomes (Briner, 1999).

Most studies which have tapped directly into general processes have been related to emotional contagion, which has

A. Vikan, *A Fast Road to the Study of Emotions*,
DOI 10.1007/978-3-319-52313-2_10

Teil I

Table 10.1 Establishing the rational environment: four ways of regulating emotions in the workplace

Neutralizing emotions
Use of routines, differentiation of roles, behavioral norms, bureaucratic practices, formalization of interactions, and distancing of relations to clients
Buffering emotion
Isolating (compartmentalizing) emotions by requiring "rational," "objective" behavior at the front-stage, and use of "detached concern" demeanor and specification of role behavior
Prescribing emotion
Role prescriptions of appropriate behavior in specific situations, masking of genuine emotions by standardized emotional expressions (e.g. smiling)
Normalizing emotion
Diffusion of emotional outbursts by apologies, remorse, and/or humor, and/or reframing them as part of a rational choice, e.g. as a manner of underlining the importance or haste of something

Based on Ashforth and Humphrey (1995)

been documented in terms of general emotional variations as "affect climate," "team climate," and "team spirit" (e.g. Abraham, 2005; Piola-Merlo, Hartel, Mann, & Hirst, 2002). Specific examples of contagion have been shown in customers who showed positive emotions and better ratings of services after displays of positive emotions in lobby tellers (Pugh, 2001), and in customers who responded both with positive emotions and positive attitude to products after display of positive emotions in salespersons (Howard & Gengler, 2001). A scale for the measurement of emotional contagion has been developed by Doherty (1997).

Contagion has also been shown to be part of leaders' influence. Two carefully designed, experimental studies where participants' emotional response were rated before and after either a task instructed individually by an actor who displayed either happiness or sadness (Barsade, 2002), or by a trained student confederate who acted either with positive or negative emotions as a leader in an in-class exercise (Bull-Schaefer & Palanski, 2013), showed emotional effects which mirrored the emotion displayed by the leader's behavior.

Another aspect of leaders' influence was shown in a study were leaders acted happy or sad in instructing an analytical and a creative task by webcan to students (Visser, van Knippenberg, van Kleef, & Wisse, 2013). The students' results were shown as better for the creative than the analytical task when the leader was happy and vice versa when he was sad, and may be conceived as dependent on participants' leader-infected emotions. This confirmed results from studies of emotional effects on cognition (see Table 6.2), and shows that leaders' emotions may influence workers' task performances through emotional contagion.

There is little else to add as regards general aspects of emotions at the workplace, but it may be noted that the emotional differences which have been associated with individualistic and collectivistic cultures (see Sect. 9.4.) are also shown in differences in organizational cultures, work-group interactions, leadership, conflict management and workplace communication (Earley & Gibson, 1998).

10.2 Emotion Work (EW)

"Emotion work" was referred to in Sect. 8.3. as emotion regulation by either surface or deep acting to comply with "feeling rules", i. e, rules or scripts for how one should act emotionally in specific situations (see Sect. 8.3). EW was directly related to the workplace in Hochschild's (1983) pivotal book as efforts to follow display rules which are stated by the administration of an organization. The rules are often stated in manuals for employees, such as Delta Airlines guide to stewards that they should be "outgoing but not effusive", "enthusiastic with calm and poise", and "vivacious but not effervescent", and show a "modest, but friendly smile" and "sincere" and "unaffected" facial expressions (op. cit. p. 96).

EW has both internal and external functions. The internal function is to establish a predictable and efficient work environment. This comprises rules that emotional outbursts should be controlled and that employees should show politeness and respect to each other and interest and concern to clients. The external function is that employees' EW advertises their firms products and policy, for instance as images of pleasantness and security. The emotional style of the offering service is in this respect a part of the service itself and shows that emotions can be a market commodity. This function is hinted at by the subheading "Commercialization of human feeling" in Hochschild's book.

Demand for EW is mainly associated with work with people. Hochschild's estimated that jobs involving a substantial emotional labor comprised 38.1% of all U.S. jobs as based on the Bureau of the Census for 1970. The jobs most calling for EW were "Professional, technical and kindred," "Managers and administrators," "Sales workers," Clerical and kindred," "Service workers excluding private household," and "Private household workers". Although many of these jobs have been automated out since 1970, this is probably more than compensated by an increase in the caring sector (childcare, nursing-homes) and in the outsourcing of family interactions and private life to, e.g. nannies, personal trainers, coaches, gift consultants, pet care assistants and birthday party planners. An example may be that the service sector comprised 59% of the European workforce at the start of the century (Zapf, 2002).

The EW approach may contribute to a realistic assessment of workloads by measuring the additional emotional work which is required in different jobs. This aim has not been obtained by the original, qualitative EW concept because EW has not been transformed into a measure which can indicate differences in amount or degree of something. When Hochschild (2003) for instance referred to studies of EW in 16 different occupations in the twentieth anniversary of her book, there were no estimates of their different emotional workloads. A definition of EW as the behavioral display of appropriate emotions (Ashforth & Humphrey, 1995) may seem better suited, but has as yet not resulted in a break-through for the approach, and neither has Brotheridge and Lee's (2003) construction of an "Emotional Labour Scale".

A more promising approach may be Morris and Feldman's (1996, 1997) proposal that EW is a process that vary in four dimensions: (1) Frequency of appropriate emotional display. (2) Attentiveness to display rules (including duration and intensity of emotional display). (3) Variety of emotions required to be displayed. (4) Emotional dissonance resulting from displaying emotions which are not genuine. The only viewpoint which links EW to the general area of emotions is Grandey (2000), who argued that EW is included in a wider process of emotion regulation which can be related to Gross' model (see Sect. 8.4).

The great merit of the EW concept is that it has served to indicate that jobs often imply an emotional workload in addition to the ordinary challenges in a job. This was implied in Hochschild's (1983) original interviews with flight attendants at Delta Airways, and has later been confirmed by findings from twelve studies that EW may result in emotional exhaustion, i.e. that employees have felt that their energy is lost and that they are drained of resources (Zapf, 2002). This effect of EW is dependent both on the job and on employee's personality. Emotional exhaustion may for instance be related to demands for EW with specific emotions, such as to hide the negative emotions of anger and fear (Brotheridge & Grandey, 2002; Naring, Vlerick, & Van de Ven, 2012), and be a more frequent result for persons with a low rather than a high ability to accept their own emotions (Biron & van Velhoven, 2012).

A main reason for EW's exhaustive effect seems to be that frequent acting of emotions (e.g. happiness) which are not genuinely felt in a particular situation results in emotional dissonance (Hulsheger & Schewe, 2011; Zapf, 2002). This induces feelings of being false and hypocritical, and includes burnout, which is a combination of emotional exhaustion, detachment towards others and a low sense of efficacy at work. Experiences of dissonance seem to be increased when employees are accused of being responsible for negative events, perceive low levels of self-accountability and do not think they are able to promote positive change (Crego, Martinez-Inigo, & Tschan, 2013).

There are, on the other hand both necessary and positive functions of EW because it maintains display rules that stabilize and standardize the work environment. This facilitates task effectiveness by regulating and making interactions predictable, and avoids embarrassing interpersonal problems that may be disruptive to work. It has, more specifically, been found in several studies that EW may be related to job satisfaction as well as to feelings of personal accomplishment (Morris & Feldman, 1997). A cause of positive results may be that interactions with others are rewarding in itself for its exchanges of behavior and viewpoints. Professional interactions may also lead to new insights in the employee, and to rewarding gratitude from clients for being helped in solving problems and satisfying needs. It even seems that EW may result in better earnings. Hulsheger, Lang, Schewe, and Zijlstra (2015) found in a study of taxi drivers, waiters and hair dressers that the amount of tips that they received for their work was related to their EW (which was called "emotion regulation" by the authors).

10.3 Emotional Intelligence (EI)

It is always a main concern of the workplace to select the best qualified recruit for each position, and it is not a new idea that the qualifications entail an understanding of other persons. It is, though, quite a recent idea that this understanding can be considered as a specifically EI. The first formal definition of EI was: "… a set of skills hypothesized to contribute to the accurate appraisal and expression of emotion, the effective regulation of emotion, and the use of feelings to motivate, plan, and achieve (Salovey & Mayer, 1989, p. 185)". The significance of EI for the workplace was interpreted to the public by Goleman (1995) in a book which became a New York Times all-time best-seller, and which has been instrumental in stimulating the emergence of a multimillion-dollar EI consulting industry and the adoption of EI-related products and services in at least 75% of Fortune 500 companies (Joseph, Jin, Newman, & O'Boyle, 2015). Research interest is indicated by the 8613 works which was listed by the PsychInfo database for a 1990–2015 search EI as a title. 32.5% 2797) of these works are recent, i.e., in 2012–2015.

Despite, or perhaps because, of this surge of interest there has been continuous doubt as to the usefulness of the concept of EI, which has been proposed as an ability parallel to conventional intelligence (Mayer, Salovey, &Caruso, 2004, 2008), as skills (Goleman, 1995a) or both as trait and ability (Petrides & Furnham, 2000, 2001). The central problem of the approach was indicated in a thorough analysis of the scientific basis of EI by the remark that "…extravagant claims as to the power of EI to predict success in the workplace appear to fly in the face of existing scientific evidence" (Matthews et al., 2005, p. 478). This is the problem of validity, which is the question whether some concept or theory is systematically related to something in the real world. The root of the problem is that EI is no single, recognizable entity but a rather fuzzy composition consisting of different components by different authors. An overview of EI components proposed in Bar-On's (2000), Goleman's (1995, 1998), and Petrides and Furnham's (2001) theories is shown in Table 10.2 (see page 72).

Table 10.2 An overview of selected EI components

Emotional self-awareness (ability to recognize and understand one's feelings)
Recognizing one's feelings and how they influence performance
Being aware of one's abilities and limitations, seeking feed-back and knowing when to work with other people
Ability to identify emotions in other people
Ability to identify clients' needs and match them to one's own products
Being aware of and appreciate others' emotions
Show astute awareness of others' emotions, concerns, and needs
Handle and manage emotions in other people and do so persuasively
Ability to express one's emotions and the needs related to them
Ability to defend one's rights in a non-destructive way
Understand and accept oneself and realize one's capacities
Believe in oneself and one's abilities
Be self-directed, self-controlled, and free of emotional dependency
Show emotional self-control and be trustworthy
Directing attention to emotionally significant stimuli
Use of emotions as an aid of thinking and memory
Ability to interpret the meanings that emotions convey
Ability to understand complex feelings or blends of feelings
Ability to stay open to emotions, both pleasant and unpleasant
Ability to reflectively detach from an emotion
Ability to monitor emotions in relation to oneself
Ability to manage emotions in oneself and others
Self-perceived ability to withstand stressful situations
Ability to read the currents of emotions and political realities in groups
Ability to establish and maintain intimate and satisfying relationships
Be a cooperative and responsible member of society
Effective in give-and-take of emotional information
Evaluate the relation between objective and subjective reality
Adjust emotions, thoughts, and behaviors to changing conditions
Withstand adverse events through positive coping
Acing before being forced by external events
Resist or delay an impulse, drive, or temptation to act
Feel satisfied with life, enjoy oneself, and enjoy being with others
Ability to spot troubles and calm those involved
Ability to inspire and guide people toward a common goal
Ability to initiate and mange change
Ability to create group synergy in pursuing collective goals

Sampled from Bar-On (2000), Goleman (1995, 1998), and Petrides and Furnham (2001)

A concept comprising the number and variation of components in 10.2 is neither viable nor meaningful. The solution is to establish reliable measurement of components which can serve to predict relevant performance (predictive validity), e.g. that applicants with a high EI score show better performance in the job in question than those with a low score. These components should also be related to each other (convergent validity) and be different from measures of other concepts (divergent validity) such as conventional intelligence and personality. Validity has been documented for several measures of EI, but there seems to be room for improvement both as regards predictive and divergent validity (Maul, 2012; Matthews et al., 2005). The main measures are Mayer, Salovey, and Caruso's (2002) Emotional Intelligence Test (MSCEIT), Bar-On's (1997) Emotional Quotient Inventory (EQ-I), Goleman's Emotional Competence Inventory (ECI) developed into ECI-2 by Boyatzis & Sala (2004), and Schutte et al.'s (1998) SSRI. A recent overview of measures is provided by Siegling, Saklofske & Petrides (2015).

Predictive validity of EI measures has most frequently been related to leadership, selection of personnel and performance of the job. The significance of leaders' ability to relate to employees and create a positive work environment has been known since the Hawthorne studies in the late 1920s (Mayo, 1933). Goleman (1998) confirmed this by referring to several studies were successful executives were shown to score much higher on EI than those who were not successful. Matthews et al. (2005) criticized Goleman's studies, but supported his evidence by referring to a study where EQ-I scores in a group of leadership achievers were much higher than in a group of chronically unemployed individuals.

The usefulness of EI for leadership seems to be confirmed by results from a majority of studies in the area. It was for instance noted in a review of studies that a relation between

EI and leadership has been demonstrated for emerging and transformational leadership, ratings of leadership potential, subordinate and managerial rankings of leadership, organizational commitment, and leader self-awareness, and that high EI leaders have been shown to achieve better business results and been rated as more effective leaders by their subordinates than by low EI leaders. Other studies have shown that high EI leaders are better able to manage conflicts and to stimulate employees' creativity than low EI leaders. Successful leadership has been specifically associated with the EI components positive moods, self-awareness and self-monitoring (Abraham, 2005). Some less than positive results have also been noted (e.g. Barbuto, Gottfredson, & Searle, 2014).

The contribution of EI to personnel selection is well established. Illiescu, Illie, Ispas and Ion (2012) showed, for instance, that measures of EI contributed to successful selection of persons to employs as salespersons, front desk public sector employees and hospital CEOs, and Joseph et al. (2015) reported in an exhaustive meta-analysis that EI showed predictive validity in relation to supervisor-rated job performance. The authors' conclusion (op. cit., p. 318) was that: "… the current results suggest that practitioners might be using measures of mixed EI as a practical, shorthand alternative to a lengthy battery of several more traditional KSAO's". It should be noted in this context that the size of differences in scores on EI tests of large groups of persons cannot automatically be generalized to selection from a small group of applicants. A difference of two points which may be predictive at the group level need, for instance, to be more than ten points to be predictive for difference in scores of two applicants. Tests of EI should therefore be supplied be information on several other indications at the personnel selection level.

EI has been shown to influence both specific and general aspects of job performance. Specific influence of EI has been related to enhanced performance (Abraham, 2005), better peer and supervisory ratings (Caruso, Bienn, & Kornacki, 2006), and low scores on burn-out. The relation of EI to general aspects of job performance has been shown as higher workplace flourishing scores, higher career adaptability, and more "organizational citizenship behavior" (Turnipseed & Vandewaa, 2012) in persons with high than with low scores on an EI measure. "Workplace flourishing" is a general indication of work engagement, satisfaction with social support and perception of power in the workplace EI, "career adaptability" is a composite of a persons' perceptions about their future and the control of their lives, curiosity about opportunities and confidence belief in the ability to cope with problems, and "organizational citizenship behavior" refers to discretionary, non-enforceable individual behaviors that has altruism and generalized compliance as the two most distinct dimensions.

Effect of EI on workplace groups is indicated by results from studies which have shown that high EI group members stimulate group functioning by higher desire of cooperation, participation, inclusion contribution to creative group decisions, and that teams with high average EI ratings have, furthermore, been found to received higher performance ratings from managers, particularly for customer service. It has even been proposed that EI might be implemented at the organizational level. Examples are, according to Abraham (2005) firms which have stimulated creativity by introducing constructive discontent, such as a debate culture (Motorola), and dissent over consensus (Sun Microsystems) to set in motion energies which might be directed into desired and productive change.

A limitation on the EI approach is that, like other approaches with a directly relevant applied aspect such as health and emotion regulation is mainly directed at emotions as a general concept. It is, for instance, not integrated into the EI approach that two persons with equal EI may have widely different emotional profiles. A person whose score refers mainly to high scores for awareness, regulation and expression of anger and fear may, for instance, be very different from another whose score refers mainly to high scores for interest and pride. Matthews et al. (2005) even held that a differentiated concept of emotions is "antithetical to the concept of EI as a general faculty" (op. cit. p. 149).

It might not do justice to the EI concept to limit the presentation to the workplace. The potential reference of this type of concept is that persons with extreme handicap in relating to emotions, such as in the autism spectrum disorders (e.g. Baron-Cohen, 1995), are critically handicapped in their ability to establish an independent personal life. This suggests that EI relates to personal adaptation as well as to cognition, which in fact was a conclusion from Petrides and Furnham's (2001) analysis of EI measures. The authors noted that some measures, e.g. the MSCEIT, referred to maximum performance in problem-solving tasks whereas others, e.g. the EQ-I, referred to typical performance as based on self-reports.

The maximum-typical distinction is a traditional one in measurement, and was interpreted by Petrides and Furnham (op. cit.) to refer to traditional cognitive abilities (maximum performance) and personality traits (typical performance). The trait interpretation relates the EI to studies of EI and health, which have shown that not only are EI associated with specific disorders such as alexithymia as well as with general life satisfaction (Austin, Saklofske, & Egan, 2005), but also, as shown in a comprehensive meta-analysis of 126 studies with responses from 19,815 participants, with mental as well as physical health (Martins, Ramalho, & Morin, 2010).

10.4 Practical Relevance

The main merit of the concepts of EW and EI may be to direct attention to the constant emotional challenges at the workplace. This should lead to measures to manage the energy which an organization has invested in its employees. EW indicates specifically a need to establish routines for emotional debriefing after exceptionally stressful episodes or periods. It is useful also to be aware of contagion both from clients, co-workers, and leaders. EI may direct to emotional learning by on the workplace by, for instance, frequent discussions about to stimulate positive energy through interest and happiness, how thinking and behavior have been or can be biased by emotional arousal, and how one's team is confronting negative and establishing positive emotional energy.

Teil I

10.5 Summary

The workplace has traditionally been considered as a rational arena where emotions have been ignored as a significant influence by the use of several suppressive mechanisms. The general emotional processes are, however, as operative in the workplace as anywhere else, as has been shown in studies of emotional contagion and emotional bias in thinking. Leaders seem to be salient factors in both these respects.

Emotions in the workplace have been especially recognized in the forms of acting designated as emotional work (EW) which often is required by employees. There are solid evidence which shows that this may represent an additional workload that is detrimental to health, and also some indication that it might be a positively stimulating.

It has also been recognized that the actors at the workplace may be different in their ability to recognize and understand emotions in themselves and others. This ability is conceived as emotional intelligence (EI), and a high EI has been shown in a large number of studies to be positive to a large variation of behavior at all levels in an organization.

Reflection Questions

1 Is your experience of effort (work) to produce happiness different from your work to control anger, sadness, or fear? In what way is the concept for this work (EW) different from the concepts of coping, emotional control and emotional regulation?

2 Which examples of emotional intelligence or lack of the same may you note from "ordinary" life (interactions at public transports, shopping, restaurants, social events, school)?

Research/Exercise Examples

1 You and your fellow students might increase your experience with EW by producing emotions such as anger, fear, and sadness according to Stanislavski's method (see Sect. 2.4).

2 An approach at measuring EI which indicates its economic significance can be to establish a scoring card for either (a) perception of responses to customers in several firms/businesses, or (b) to score the response from an employee when you ask for information and make a negative comment on products. The scores should be (e.g.) for the degree on a five-point scale that the employee greets you, show attention, listen adequately, display positive feeling, responds seriously, show patience, and ends the interaction in a polite way. You should also score your impression after the interaction in term of the degree to which you would feel (a) or felt (b) respected, appreciated and taken seriously, as well as the degree to which you would want to buy something from the employee, to return to the employee for advice and possible to buy something afterwards, and to talk well about the employee and recommend the employee to your friends and your family. You should also score your happiness, anger, and sadness in each instance.

Which co-variations of factors or cause-effect relations might be suggested in the results from this type of study?

Further Reading

Goleman, D. (1995). *Emotional intelligence. Why it can matter more than IQ*. London: Bloomsbury.

Hochschild, A. R. (2003). *The managed heart. The commercialization of human feeling*. Berkeley: The University of California Press.

Mayer, J. D., Salovey, P., & Caruso, D. R. (2008). Emotional intelligence: New ability or eclectic traits? *American Psychologist, 63,* 503–517.

Historical Background and Current Theories

11

Something called emotions was mentioned in Greek philosophy, but emotions as we know them were probably not a subject of discussions before early in the eighteenth century. Concepts of emotions before this time may have been blends of what is now called need, desire, passion, affect, and will. The focus when emotions were discussed was on the distinction between pleasant and unpleasant experiences, which is a dimension that has been the main criterion for the classification of emotions until Russell and Feldman Barretts' modern theory (see Sect. 11.3.2). Reflections on qualitative differences between emotions are not known before Spinoza's philosophical discussions of the logic of love and hate in «The Ethic» in 1677.

This chapter starts with a short note on reflections on emotions in classical philosophy, and proceeds to a note on Darwin (1872), whose use of scientific method to study emotions and his report on the results of his studies in (1872) can be counted as the starting point for a science of emotions. This is followed by a note on the James-Lange physiological theory of emotions and Wundts theory of dimensions of emotional experience in the 1890s, and Watson and Cannon's views non emotion in first part of the 20th Century. Modern research on emotions is set to a two-fold focus on a cognitive and a neo-Darwinian biological approach in 1954, the description in chapter notes the highlights of this research till about 1990, which represent a time for a marked increase in the amount and diversity of emotion research.

The last part of this chapter is short descriptions of three current theories. Two of these, Izard's differential emotions- and Russell and Feldman Barretts' dimensional theory, held that emotions originates in neurobiological activity, the former assumes that this is a core which is extended to emotions in interaction with cognition, and the latter that emotions are a result of classification of experience related to social categories. The third theory is Oatley & Johnson-Lairds information science theory that emotions are actually coordinated information from different cognitive modules that serve to organize the organism's resources and direct to relevant action.

11.1 Philosophical Background

Modern studies on emotions were preceded by philosophy and by a general development of science at the end of the 19th Century. The start of the known inquiries within philosophy seems to be Democritus (500 f.Kr.), but it was Plato (428–348 f.Kr.) and Aristotle (384–322) who did the first analyzes. Both philosophers, as was noted in Chap. 6, considered emotions as threats to reason. Aristotle recognized that emotions as central to human life, and knew that they were associated both with cognition and physiological reactions. He held that emotions resulted from what we perceive and think, i.e. cognition, and that they must be regulated. Thus, he reflected that we must show suitable affect in suitable situations if we are not to be considered fools (Aristotle, 2000). The stoic philosophers' valuation of moderation and control was a main principle in the classic Greek thinking and relation to emotions. This also comprised epicureans' viewpoints, and became an ideal to Roman culture. The stoics classified emotions into the four basic "agitations" sadness, happiness, fear, and desire (Lyons, 1992; Oatley, 2004; Oatley & Jenkins, 1996; Strongman, 1996).

There was little development in the thinking about emotions before Descartes (1596–1650) and Spinoza (1632–1677) in the 17th Century. Descartes followed Aristotle in proposing that emotions result from cognitions and consist of physiological reactions which move the soul because they refer to something which is important. This shows the dualism between body and soul, or soma or psyche, which has been dominant in Western thinking until this day. Descartes proposed that emotions were based in the brain, specifically the pineal gland. These viewpoints actually comprised three major parts of modern research on emotions: Cognition, physiological reactions, and localization of emotions to the brain.

Spinoza's reflections on emotions were focused on passions. Passions were conceived of as managing our responses and choices. Spinoza proposed that we can obtain freedom from the passions by learning how to control them. This can be done by being conscious of their causes. He tried to provide support for persons who wanted to gain conscious control by elaborate analyses of specific passions, notably hate and love.

A. Vikan, *A Fast Road to the Study of Emotions*,
DOI 10.1007/978-3-319-52313-2_11

11.2 Introductory Studies and Viewpoints: Darwin, James and Wundt

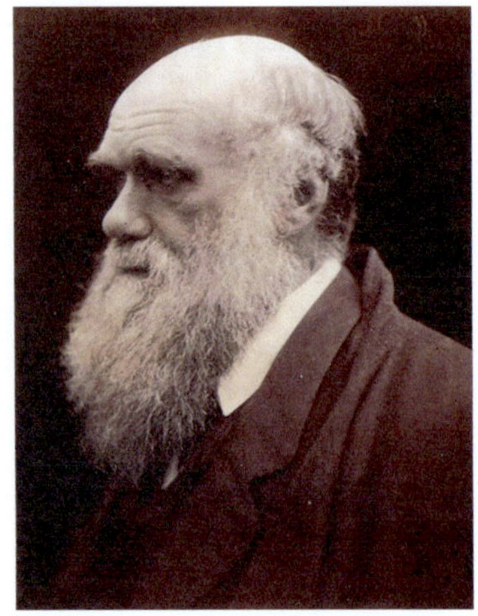

Picture 11.1 Charles Darwin (1809–1882)

Charles Darwin (1809–1882) Picture 11.1 was a biologist and is historically dominating to the extent that he can be held as the founder of the science of emotions. His viewpoints were related to his well-known theory of natural selection and the proposition that emotional expressions are based on neurological circuits. The main point for the development of a science was, however, that his viewpoints were based on evidence from scientific method. Darwin (1872) did not define emotions in his book on emotions in animals and man from, and did not differentiate clearly between the expression of emotions and emotions as a phenomenon. His theoretical viewpoints were cited in Sects. 1.5, 2.2, 2.3, 2.5 and 9.4. We have also referred to his method, which

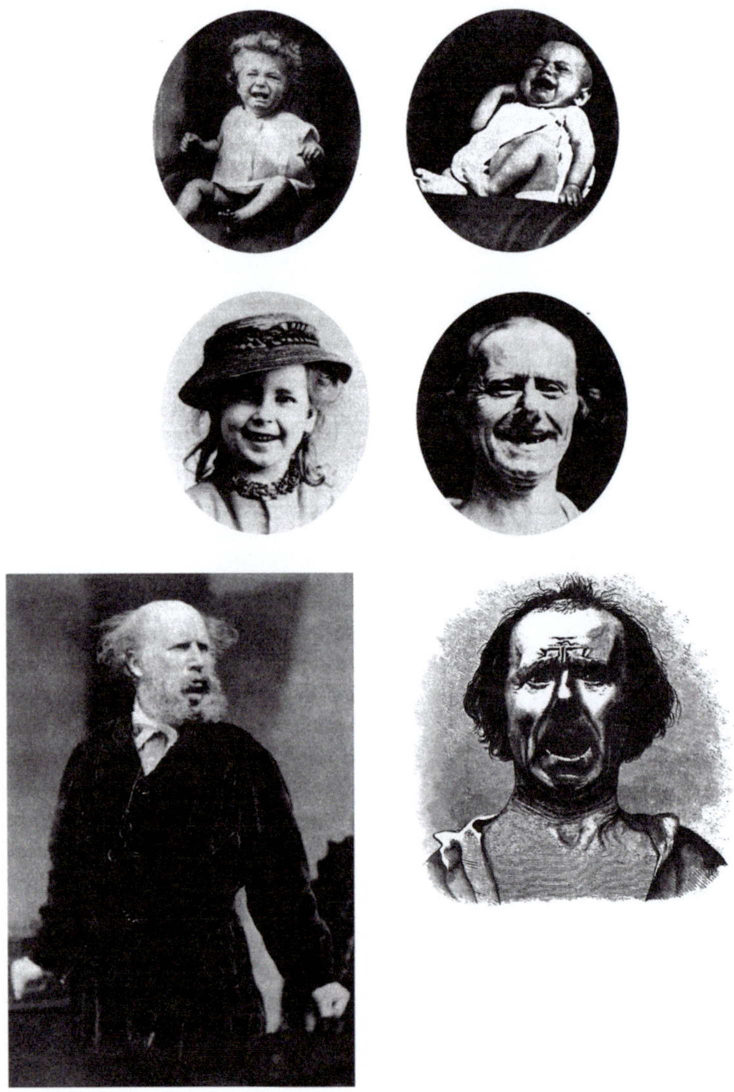

Fig. 11.1 Photographs used as illustrations by Darwin (1872) showing happiness (*upper row*), sadness (*middle row*), anger (*low row left*), and fear (*low row right*)

consisted of the use of drawings, photos and interviews in addition to a great many observations from daily life, including children's behavior. Darwin even got access to a mental hospital in order to observe expressions of emotions in the patients. His use of questionnaire to missionaries at different places in the world (see Sect. 2.6) was pioneering both for the questionnaire method and for cross-cultural comparisons. Examples of photographs used by Darwin are shown in Fig. 11.1 (see page 76).

William James (1842–1910) was a North American philosopher who is part of the history of studies on emotions because of his textbook on psychology in 1890 where he argued that emotions are the experience of physiological reactions. A very similar concept was proposed five years earlier by the Danish physiologist Carl Lange, and the theory is now known as the James-Lange theory of emotions. The standard example is that fear is the experience of physiological signals when a person is fleeing from danger, e.g. an angry dog. The emotional experiences (cognition) was, consequently, assumed to be caused by the physiological reactions, in contradistinction to the common view that physiological reactions and emotional experiences are caused by cognition of a stimulus or an event, as was shown in Lazarus and Alfert's (1964) study in Sect. 6.1.1 and indicated by the model of emotional causation in Sect. 1.6.

Wilhelm Wundt (1832–1929) was a medical doctor who became the founder of scientific psychology. Wundt considered emotions as a main part of consciousness, and held that emotional experiences could be classified in relation to the dimensions pleasure-unpleasure, excitement-suppression (control), and excitations-relaxation.

11.3 Modern Research on Emotions

11.3.1 Before 1950: Watson, Cannon and Research on the Brain

The study of emotions stagnated in the first half of the 20th Century. The most marked contribution was the behaviorist Watson's (1878–1958) demonstration that an 11 month old child could learn to fear something (a rat) which he did not fear initially. This supported a concept of emotions as learned behavior (Watson & Raynor, 1920).

The physiologist Walter Cannon (1871–1945) pioneered physiological and neurological studies of emotions. Cannon is known, in addition to the identification of emotional crisis reactions which were referred in Sect. 7.4, for a test of the James-Lange theory where he injected persons with adrenaline in order to speed up their physiological responses. The physiology was speeded up, but the results were negative, there were no reports on the emotions expected from the James-Lange theory (Cannon, 1927).

Experiments on animals and studies of functional problems related to neurological damage were well under way in the 20s and 30s. A result of this was that the Nobel Price in medicine was awarded to the Swiss Walter Hess and the Portuguese Egas Moniz in 1949. Hess had developed electrodes which could be implanted in the brain, and showed that emotional behavior could be directly triggered by electrical stimulation in specific areas (e.g. the hypothalamus). Moniz was awarded the price because he had shown that lesions in the frontal lobe in humans ("lobotomization") led to an elimination of aggression.

11.3.2 1950s: Cognitive Revolution and Rediscovery of Darwin

Modern scientific research on emotions is often set to 1954, when Magda Arnold (1903–2002) Picture 11.2 and Silvan Tomkins (1911–1991) Picture 11.3 published their theories.

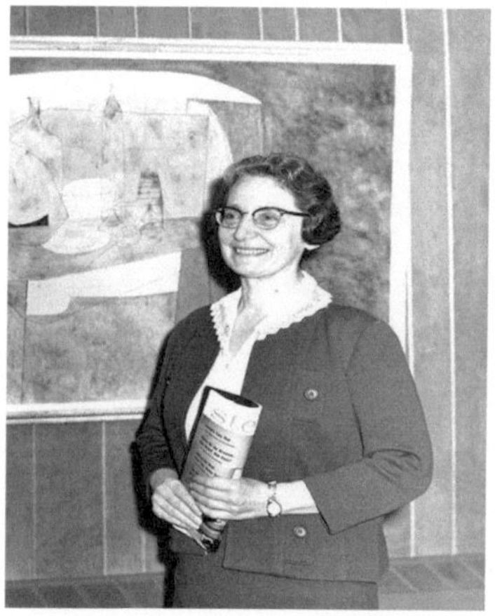

Picture 11.2 Magda Arnold (1903–2002)

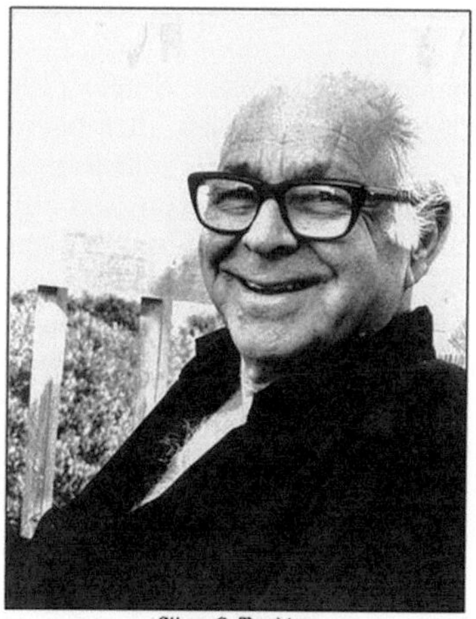

Picture 11.3 Silvan Tomkins (1911–1991)

Arnold argued in an article this year that emotions are results of appraisal of whether something is positive or negative (see Arnold, 1968). This is the foundation of appraisal theories of emotions (see Sect. 6.1). Tomkins' (1962, 1963) theories were based on Darwin's assumptions that emotions relate to neurological circuits and are part of the facial expressions (see Sects. 1.2 and 2.2).

One of Tomkins' original ideas was that emotions functions as amplifiers when they are aroused. Amplifying is theorized to mobilize neuronal and physiological support to co-ordinate reactions into a specific emotion at the same time as it attenuate stimuli and/or events in the surroundings which are important for this emotions. This, in addition to a concept of emotions as motivational systems (see Sect. 1.2) and a differentiation between drives and emotions, posed "emotions" as a clear and independent subject of study. A main argument for the differentiation of drives and emotion was that drives function according to a sequence represented by arousal, satisfaction, and termination which is different from emotional functioning, which is not characterized by a specific termination.

11.3.3 1960–1980. Schachter and Singer, Richard Lazarus (1922–2002), Paul Ekman (B. 1934) and Carroll Izard (1923–2017)

There were two centers of gravity for the study of emotions which developed in a fruitful 20–30 years period from 1960. The first was cognitive, inspired by Arnold and was influenced and reinforced by a breakthrough of cognitive analyses following the development of feed-back control mechanisms, information technology, and Chomsky's linguistic theory. The significance of cognition was demonstrated by Lazarus and Alfert's study (1964) which was described in Sect. 6.1. The first "cognitive" study on emotions was, however, conducted by Stanley Schachter and Jerome Singer (1962). Participants in the study rated their emotions after having been aroused physiologically by an adrenalin injection and placed in a situation where another person expressed either happiness or anger. The results showed that the participants' highest emotional rating was the emotion which corresponded to that of the other person. The results were interpreted as showing that arousal is necessary for an emotional experience in general, but that it is the cognition (of the other person) which determines the experience of a specific emotion.

The other center of gravity in the time period was a follow-up on inspirations from Darwin and Tomkins by Ekman's and Izard's studies (see Sects. 2.5 and 9.3). Ekman's contribution is focused on the universality and analysis of facial expressions, whereas Izard is focused on children's emotions, emotion–cognition interactions, and the characterization of individual emotions.

11.3.4 The 80S and 90S and Further. Bower, Zajonc and Isen

A further and even more salient focus on cognition followed in the steps of Gordon Bower (b. 1932) and Robert Zajonc (1923–2008) , who were awarded APA's price for excellence in research in, respectively, 1980 and 1981. The best known results from these studies are probably the support for Bower's congruence hypothesis, which was cited in Sect. 6.2.1 and was illustrated by Fig. 6.1. Zajonc received the price for research results which were interpreted as showing that emotions do not need to be based on appraisals because they are directly given in the experience. An example used in Zajonc's argumentation was that we often remember that we have preferred or disliked something without knowing any causes of this. These ideas were strongly contested by Lazarus in an important discussion where he argued that emotions are dependent on cognition against Zajonc's view that emotions, in terms of "affects", are primary and based on a separate system in the brain.

Alice Isen (1942–2012) pioneered the study of positive emotions. She had already conducted studies which showed that happiness led to increased helpfulness in 1970 (Isen & Levin, 1972). A series of studies which showed the effects of happiness which were cited in Sect. 6.2.4 were conducted in the early 1980s.

Modern research on emotions was well established in the 1990s. Central contributions to the area around this date was delivered by Oatley and Johnson-Laird (1987) , Ortony, Clore, and Collins (1988), Frijda (1986), Scherer (1988), Izard (1991) , Lazarus (1991) , MacLean (1990), Panksepp (1991), LeDoux (1991) and Damasio (1994). The research results and theories from these authors confirmed the cognitive approach, but the biological approach gained momentum by the new methods in studies of activity in the brain, i.e. the functional neuroimaging (fMRI) and the position emission tomography (PET) techniques (see Sect. 1.4).

Research on emotions the last 20 years has many-sided to the extent that it is difficult to render an integrated and exhaustive description. Major areas and subjects have been or will be presented in this book, such as cross-cultural studies, neuropsychological studies (Chap. 12), and studies on stress and coping, emotion regulation, positive emotions and emotional intelligence. The practical use of knowledge about emotions has increased on a broad basis. The main theme has been the treatment of mental health problems, but new approaches are made in relation to physical health, child care, organizational behavior and interaction at the work-place, training and instructions for teams and individual performers and in relation to learning in the schools. Table 11.1 (see page 79) provides an overview on the historical background.

Table 11.1 Historical overview on research on emotions

Time period key words for persons and themes
Philosophers Plato and Aristotle. Emotions as disturbance
400 B. C. of reason
Philosophers Descartes: Emotions move the soul
17 Century Spinoza: Emotions are passions which can be controlled by consciousness
End of Darwin: Emotions in the brain, development of
19th Century scientific studies. James: Emotions are experiences of physiological reactions. Wundt: Three dimensions in the experience of emotions
1910–1930 Watson showed that fear can be learned, Cannon described crisis reactions and argued against the James-Lange theory
1950 Arnold initiated appraisal theory, Tomkins rediscovered Darwin and described emotions as motivational systems
1960 Schachter & Singer and Lazarus with studies which showed that emotions results from cognition
1970 Ekman and Izard conducted studies with results which indicated that facial expressions are universal
1980 Bower and Isen with studies of emotions' influence on cognition and positive emotions,respectively, Zajonc argued that emotions need no preferences
1990 New theories, modern neuroscience into emotions, *and further* emotions and health, positive emotions, emotional intelligence, and emotion regulation

11.4 Modern Theoretical Approaches

The different influences on-, and variations in components of emotions have, according to Griffin and Mascolo (1998) inspired five different frames for theories on emotion: (a) Biologically based theories, (b) Cognitive approaches, (c) Developmentally structured theories, (d) Functionalistic approaches, and (e) Sociocultural theories. This comprises a large number of theories. Strongman (1996) referred, for instance, to 76 different theoretical viewpoints in his book on the subject (see also Plutchik, 1980; Turner & Stets, 2005).

New theories usually include previous ones. Most of previous theories are, therefore, represented in the three modern theories which are presented in this book: Izard's biologically based, Russell and Feldman Barrett's dimensional-, and Oatley and Johnson-Laird's cognitive theory.

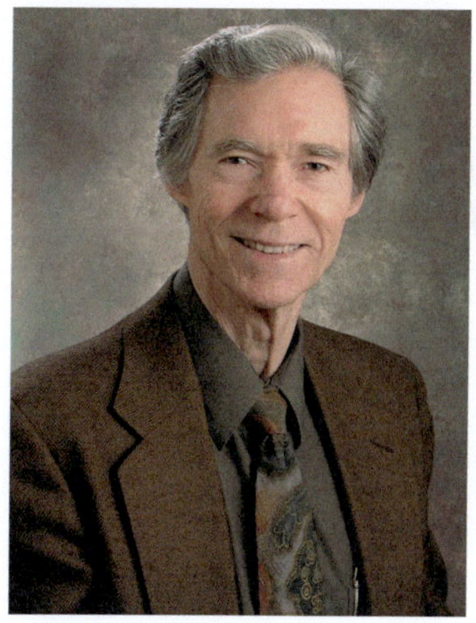

Picture 11.4 Carroll Izard (1923–2017)

11.4.1 Carroll E. Izard and Differential Emotion Theory

Izard's (Picture 11.4) theory is built on Tomkins' conception that emotions comprise a primary motivational system, are formed in the evolution and are neural structures which are determined and expressed via facial expressions. The neural structures are assumed to comprise a program for a sample of basic emotions which are differentiated in terms of qualities of experiences, expression, and motivational directions and goals. The basic emotions are also characterized by being present at, or a short time after birth with a motor, or neuromuscular component, imply regulations that influence cognition and behavior, show very fast processing of information, have short duration and are primed to react to specific stimuli (for instance a fire or a snake) (Ackerman, Abe, & Izard, 1998; Izard, 2007, 2009; Izard & Ackerman, 2000). "Basic" in this context does not mean that the emotions are functionally "independent" or "discrete", emotions in differential emotions theory are all conceived as interacting and mutually influencing parts in an emotional system (Izard, 1971, 1972).

The ten basic emotions in Table 1.3 were modified to six in the most recent discussion (Izard, 2009) . Surprise was out of the list because it was reconsidered as part of interest, and shame, guilt, and contempt was excluded because there are not shown any universal facial expressions for these emotions. Izard emphasized interest as a normative and primary emotion because it functions at a level of intensity which is necessary for conscious experience, and because it serves as an entrance to other emotions via attention. Arousal of emotions was related to four different systems: Neural, sensation-motor, affective-motivational, and cognitive (Izard, 1993). Emotions may, for instance, be aroused by psychoactive drugs and direct stimulation of the brain (neural), by muscles in the face and bodily stance (sensation-motor), by smell, taste, and other emotions (affective-motivational), and by appraisals (cognitive).

The starting point for emotions is, according to Izard, an "emotion feeling". This was conceived as a phase in neurobiological activity which signals that something is important to the organism. Neurobiological activity is comprised of integrated activity from the brain stem, the amygdala, the insula, the anteriorfrontal cingulate and the orbifrontal cortices (see Chap. 12). This activity is assumed to include different emotion feelings in the same way as different colors are included in the visual system. Emotion feeling is also assumed to comprise both motivation and information functions. This can be the content of an "early warning system" (see Sect. 1.4) where emotion feeling serves as an algorithm for the relation to the surroundings and for the organization of responses. The emotion feeling is held to turn into a basic emotion when information from the neurobiological activity reaches the experience (i.e. is integrated in neural stimulation which form an experience).

Izard (2007) held that basic emotions are very infrequent when the child is three-four years of age because they are then linked to a cognitive development which started right after birth. The "linking" or "integration" of emotion and cognition was held to form "schemas" Schemas represent connections between components of emotion feelings, memories and experiences which may seem similar to the emotion congruent memories hypothesized as the reasons of the results in Bower's studies (see Sect. 6.2.1). All the basic emotions can, according to Izard (2007), be integrated into schemas and form "schema emotions". It can be suggested that "schema emotions" is a parallel to what has been called "ordinary emotions" in this book (see Sect. 5.1), and represents an opening of social, cognitive and cultural influence on emotions.

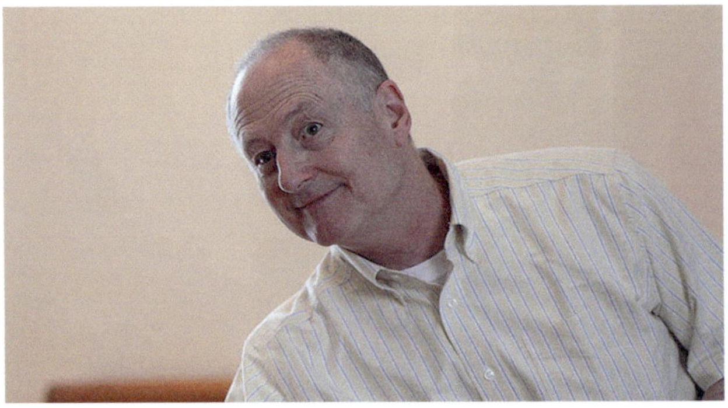

Picture 11.5 James Russell (b. 1947)

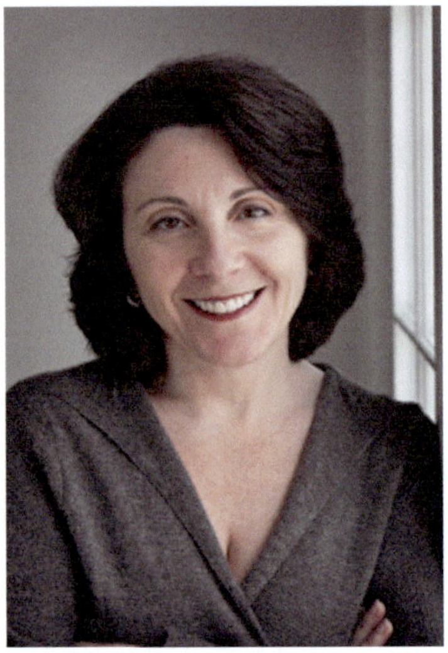

Picture 11.6 Lisa Feldman Barrett (b. 1963)

11.4.2 James A. Russell and Lisa Feldman Barrett: Dimensions and Cognitive Constructs

James Russell and Lisa Feldman Barrett's (respectively pictures 11.5 and 11.6) theory is based on studies of classification of emotional experiences. This is done by having participants rate each emotion in relation to various characteristics. The procedure is similar to the search for dimensions of meaning and appraisal which were described in, respectively, Sects. 4.1 and 6.1.2. Statistical analyses on a very large number of ratings have repeatedly resulted in the identification of two dimensions, valence (pleasant-unpleasant) and arousal (activation-deactivation). This means that the meaning a person associates with a specific emotion is influenced bidimensionally by a valence scale from very positive to very negative, and from an arousal scale from intensely activated to deactivated. This is indicated by the structure of meaning shown in Fig. 11.2 (see page 81) (Feldman Barrett & Russell, 1998). Figure 11.2 means, for instance, that sadness is felt as a strongly unpleasant and mildly to strongly passive emotion and happiness as a very pleasant and mildly to strongly activating emotion. Other emotions, such as fear, will be between tense and nervous and be felt as very unpleasant and very activating, and anger will be between stressed and upset and felt about as unpleasant as fear, but somewhat less activating (Feldman Barrett & Russell, 1998).

Note that Russell and Feldman Barrett's dimensional descriptions form a contrast to the qualitative differentiations of individual emotions in Izard's differential emotions theory. The point of departure is, however, not very different. It is hypothesized in Russell and Feldman Barrett's theory that emotions are rooted in a core affect conceived as a neurophysiological state which is a biological product of the evolution. The state is assumed to be part of a continuous stream of homeostatic feedback varying in valence and activation from the body. The significance is that the core affect functions as a neurophysiological barometer for a person's relation to the surroundings (Feldman Barrett, 2005; Russell, 2003).

Variations in core affect are assumed to result in feelings of being moved, forced/influenced and/or being generally emotional. But there is yet no experience of an emotion. This

Fig. 11.2 Dimensions of emotional experience. The letters *x* and *y* represent meaning components: *x* pleasantness; *y* activation (from Feldman Barrett & Russell, 1998)

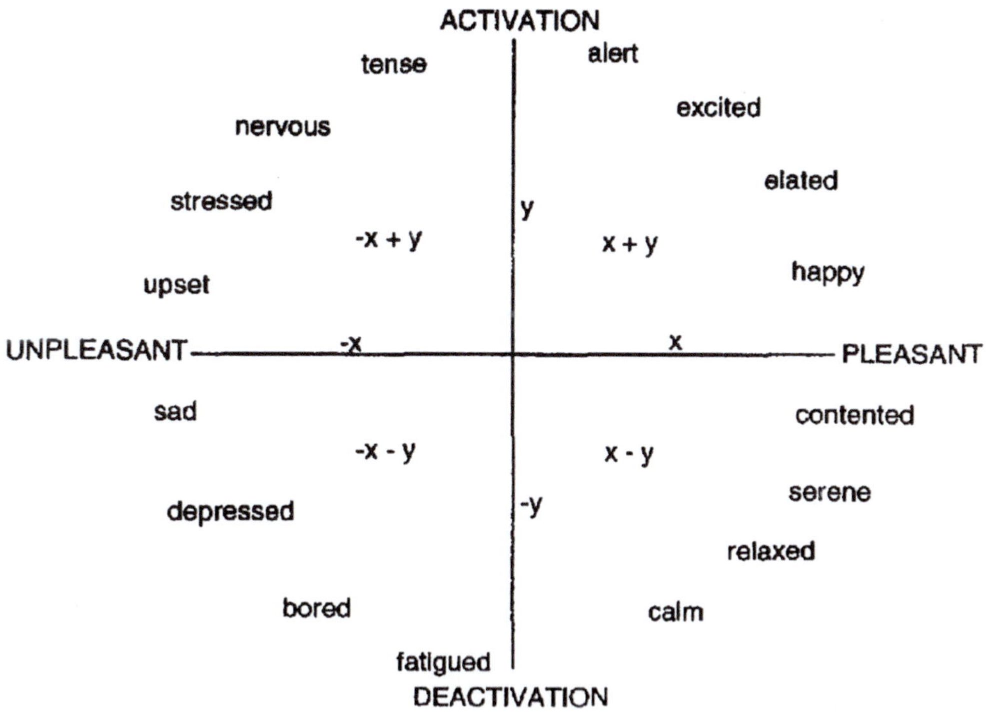

experience is beginning to form when the core affect is attributed to a some cause, and is developed as an emotion when the person recognizes her/his reactions as corresponding to reactions which is described by a specific emotion word in the social environment. The experience has at that point become sufficiently distinct to be named. Emotions are, according to the theory, rough categorizations of experiences. The categories are held to comprise recipes for different types of emotions in terms of physiological changes, behavior, vocalizations and facial expressions, in addition to social rules for the behavioral expression (Feldman Barrett, 2005).

The theory implies that emotions are definitively not the "natural kinds" which are envisaged in Izard's (2007) biologically oriented theory. Emotions in Russell and Feldman Barrett's theory are something that can vary with type of society and culture, and Russell (1994) has, consequently, been very critical of Ekman's and Izard's cross-cultural studies. But the anchoring of emotions to the neurophysiological core affect shows that the theory does not imply an interpretation of emotions as mere constructions (Russell, 2003).

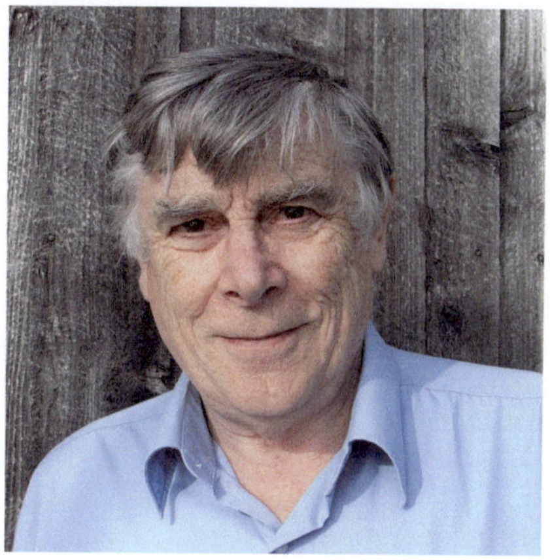

Picture 11.7 Keith Oatley (b. 1937)

11.4.3 Keith Oatley and Philip Johnson-Laird: Adjustment to Cognitive Science

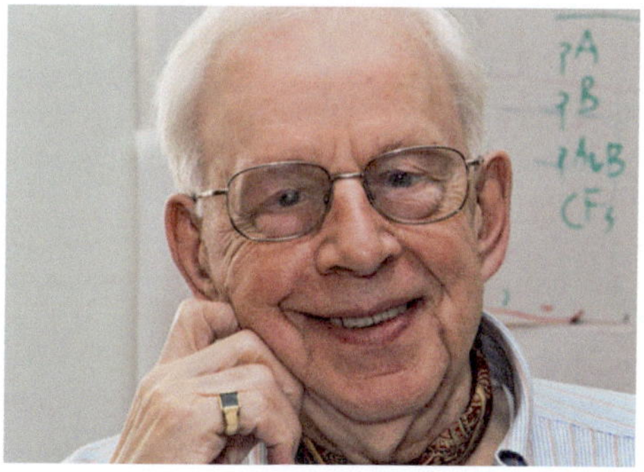

Picture 11.8 Philip Johnson-Laird (b. 1936)

Oatley and Johnson-Laird's (OJL) (respectively pictures 11.7 and 11.8) theory of emotions (Oatley & Johnson-Laird, 1987)

Teil I

Table 11.2 Key words for three theoretical views on emotions

	Izard	Russell and Feldman Barrett	Oatley and Johnson-Laird
Initial state	Phase in neurobiological activity	Neurobiological state	Challenge to organism
Basic form	Emotion feeling	Core affect	Coordinated info. from cognitive modules
Basic experience	Exp. of activity	Exp. of being moved, perc. of influence	Exp. of coord. module signals
First emotions	Basic emotion	Attribution of causation to movement/influence	Conscious appraisal of coord. info.
Further development	Coordination emotion-cognition	Linking causal attribution & social category for emotion	Basic emotion
Developed form	Schema-emotions	Categorization of experience by emotion names	Blended and extended emotions

is an attempt to harmonizing the study of emotions and cognitive science. The great contribution assumed to follow is that harmonizing provides a solution to the central problem in modern data systems and artificial intelligence according to Simon (1967) that the they do not include a directional advice about how to proceed when a program is interrupted. There will be lots of available programs in this case, but no background for priorities in such «cold» systems. Emotions are the solution to the problem because they motivate to new goals which imply a selection of further activity.

The point of departure for the theory is cognitive, and is an assumption that cognition is organized in sub-systems of modules. A module is seen as an independent unit with a goal. Getting up in the morning and having breakfast are, for instance, examples of two different modules with two different goals. Modules are assumed to function by sending signals related to a problem or a challenge (need, wish). The signals from different modules are hypothesized to be coordinated, and it is this coordination which is considered as the content of emotions. The experience of happiness when one is about to go to the school or to work in the morning is, for instances, a coordination of the getting-up and eating-breakfast modules. The coordination is assumed to function via communication signals which set the modules for specific types of organization.

It is, furthermore, proposed that emotional signals from the coordination spread rapidly in the cognitive system and lead to a control, for instance when one want something. Coordination may, in fact, be a concept that corresponds to Izard's concept of emotion feeling, and to Russell and Feldman Barratt's concept of core affect as a "barometer" of the body's functioning. OJL theorized that the signals follow non-specific trajectories in order to trigger a quick response because they are stimulated by peptides or chemical influence. The meeting point between the modules represents a modus which prepares for action in specific directions. This is seen as a necessary, but not a sufficient condition for an emotion. An emotion is not considered as developed before a person is able to appraise a meeting point from the different modules because it is this which can ascribe a meaning that selects a direction for behavior.

It is the preparation for action in the meeting points, I.e. the emotion, which is conceived as the solution to Simon's (1967) problem. OJL emphasize that this represents a biological solution to the challenge of how to plan and perform to attain goals in an unforeseeable environment. This requires a set-up which is much more flexible than the specific and detailed programs which have been designed in studies of artificial intelligence. Oatley and Jenkins (1996) suggested that the content of the emotion modus are simple inferences of what has happened and how to respond. This means that emotions are conceived as simplifications and heuristics which can be applied in situations without a defined solution.

Happiness, anger, sadness, fear, and disgust are regarded by OJL as basic modes. The only characteristic noted for the basic modes is that they comprise universal facial expressions. Surprise and interest are regarded as including several emotions and are not conceived as basic. Others, such as jealousy or resentment, are considered as extensions of basic emotions by being attributed new meanings. An overview of basic concepts in the three theories is presented in Table 11.2.

11.5 Summary

The study of emotions has historical roots to Greek philosophy, where emotions were conceived as disturbances of reason that can be controlled, and as resulting in part from cognition (Aristotle, Plato). They were interpreted in modern philosophy in the 17th Century by Descartes, who proposed that emotions moves the soul and result from cognition, and by Spinoza, who regarded emotions as forces which we could use provided that we became conscious of their causes.

The first scientific study of emotions was inspired by Charles Darwin, William James og Wilhelm Wundt. Darwin has influences subsequent research by designing methods for concrete studies and by theories that emotions are universal, inherited and manifested in facial expressions. William James provoked discussions and testing with a theory, preceded by Carl Lange, that emotional experience is the result of physiological changes, and Wilhelm Wundt proposed three dimensions in emotional experience.

Emotions were almost ignored until the 1950s. Watson had by then demonstrated that fear can be learned (around 1915), and Cannon in the 1920s and 1930s had confronted the

James-Lange theory, described crisis reactions and opened the study of physiological and neurological bases of emotions.

Magda Arnold proposed in the 1950s that emotions are results of appraisal, and was followed up by Schachter Schachter and Singer and Lazarus in the 60s, and by Bower, Zajonc and Isen in the 80s. This represented a break-through for cognitive psychology in the interpretation of emotions. A parallel force in the study of emotions until the present has been extensions of Tomkins', Izard's and Ekman's rediscovery of Darwin's biologically based, evolutionistic views on emotions.

Izard's theory of emotions is in part an extension of Tomkins' and Darwin's viewpoints, and comprises an emotional feeling rooted in neurobiological activity which results in six inherited, basic emotions differentiated in terms of qualities of experience, expression, and motivation. Basic emotions are assumed to combine with cognition and result in schema emotions.

Russell and Feldman Barrett developed a theory related to a concept of emotions as resulting from common classifications of the experience of emotional experiences and their causes, and a classification of emotions related to the dimensions valence and activation.

Emotions in Oatley & Johnson-Lairds theory are conceived as the product of a challenge to the organism which provokes a coordination of information from different cognitive modules and which results in an organization of resources and relevant action.

Reflection Questions

1. The history which is described in this chapter starts with Charles Darwins' 1872 book, although emotions have been explored in many centuries before that time. Why should Darwin be given the honor as a founder of emotional science?
2. Whereas Feldmann Barrett and Russell strongly argue that emotions vary along two dimensions, Izard's differential emotions theory imply that emotions vary qualitatively in terms of different types. Are these viewpoints reciprocally excluding, or can one be included in the other?

Research/Exercise Examples

1. You should read at least one chapter of Darwin's book "The expression of the emotions in man and animals".
2. It may be assumed that the focus has been on a few basic negative emotions (fear, anger, and sadness) during the history of emotion research. You can test the assumption by noting the frequency of different types of emotions in the title of scientific publications each tenth or twentieth year from 1900 to 2015. Can you hypothesize that there is any shift in relative frequencies during this time?

Further Reading

Darwin, C. (1872). *The expression of the emotions in man and animals*. London: Albemarle.

Izard, C. E. (2009). Emotion theory and research: Highlights, unanswered questions, and emerging issues. *Annual Review of Psychology, 60,* 1–25.

Oatley, K. (2004). *Emotions. A brief history*. Oxford: Blackwell.

Russell, J. A. (2003). Core affect and the psychological construction of emotion. *Psychological Review, 110,* 145–172.

Strongman, K. T. (1996). *The Psychology of emotion. Theories of emotion in perspective* (4th ed.). New York: John Wiley & Sons.

12 Biological Basis of Emotions

The first part of this chapter is a review of the anatomical and neuronal mapping with lateralization and the amygdala as main themes and with reference to the theory that fear can be triggered both from a "fast and dirty" subcortical, and a slower, cortical road via thalamus to the amygdala. A contrasting viewpoint is cited that the amygdale mainly is an integrating function which also handles information from vision via the visual cortex and from cognition via the hippocampus. Information on other emotions than fear was scarce before fMRI and PET scanning have indicated associations of several parts of the brain with happiness, sadness, and anger.

The last part of the chapter is devoted to a description of the physiological basis of emotional responses. This implies some repetition about the function of the ANS, and comprises a review of research and discussions about the specificity of emotional reactions I.e. whether each emotion shows a specific physiological reaction pattern. There are indications of several specific differences for anger, fear, sadness, disgust, and happiness, but conclusions from recent reviews of research is that the only robust differences are between ANS-activation of positive and negative emotions. This chapter closes with a short note on neurochemical influences on emotion.

12.1 Anatomical and Neuronal Basis of Emotions

A well-known demonstration of the relationship of the brain to psychological functioning is the fate of the railroad foreman Phineas Gage, who got a 2 m and 6 kg iron rod by an explosion accident into his left eye, through his left frontal lobe (see Fig. 12.1, page 86) and out through the top of his skull in September 1848. Gage survived to live another 12 years, but his personality including his emotional responses, were profoundly changed.

Brain damaged patients and animal studies have traditionally been the most important sources of information about the relation between the brain and emotions. A special reason for the use of animals is that emotions have a background in the evolutionary old, subcortical part of the brain. The subcortical part regulates the physiological functions and the basic orientation to the surrounding world, is dominant in animals and is common to animals and humans. An overview of the subcortical parts is shown in Fig. 1.4. The new part of the brain (the cortex) is developed in humans, and is the basis for higher mental functions, such as abstract thinking, long time planning and language. The cortex has four main areas called "lobes" separated by fissures. The four lobes are shown on top of the spinal cord and the cerebellum in Fig. 12.1, which also shows the parts of the cortex that sends information to the muscles (the somatomotor cortex) and detects and interpret information from the senses (somatosensory cortex).

Each of the lobes is a main area for psychological functions. The most important is the frontal, which comprises 1/3 of the cortex and is the area for thinking (e.g. planning and reasoning), spoken language and motor functions. The injury suffered by Phineas Gage was in the frontal lobe and was, typically, shown as a loss of planning capacity and emotional control. The parietal lobe comprises areas for touch and understanding of language, the occipital lobe comprises information to visual perception, and the temporal lobe comprises information for audition and memory (by connection to the hippocampus).

Many researchers have assumed that our common subcortical brain means that results from studies on animals are valid also for humans. Studies were initially been made by opening the animals' brains and stimulate various brain areas electrically or chemically. Modern research has been able to use learning as indications of the brain's functional characteristics, for instance in combination with masking techniques such as in Øhman and Soares (1994) and Dimberg, Thunberg, and Elmehed (2000) studies, which were cited in, respectively, Sects. 1.7 and 2.6. The traditional method for studies on humans has been the electroencephalogram (EEG). The EEG consists of having electrodes fastened to the skull to register brain activity in terms of electrical signals. The method is now exchanged to a large extent by the modern fMRI and PET neuroimaging techniques (see Sect. 1.4).

A. Vikan, *A Fast Road to the Study of Emotions*,
DOI 10.1007/978-3-319-52313-2_12

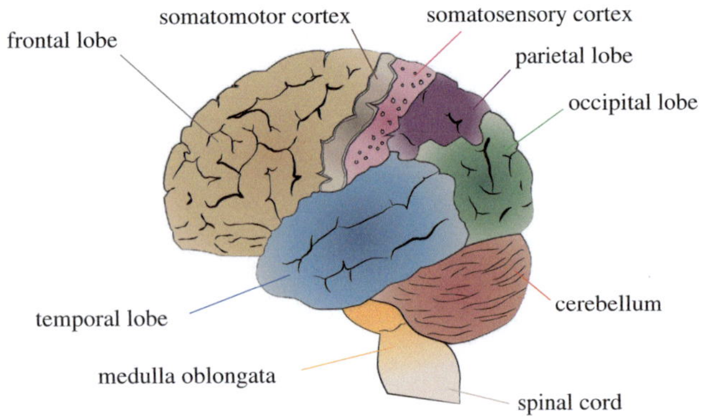

Fig. 12.1 Overview of the cortex (from Blausen com.staff. "Blausen gallery 2014")

12.1.1 Lateralization

The brain consists of two halves with different functions. This is called "lateralization", and means that the main foundation for emotions is in the right half of the brain, whereas the left half is the background for language and thought. Studies of the functions of the different halves can be made by paralyzing one of the halves while the other is tested with some task. A picture shown with the left half paralyzed will, for instance, result in emotional reactions, while the same picture shown with the right half paralyzed leads to logical thought and meaning related to the theme on the picture. Lateralization is also shown in terms of different characteristics. Persons with a dominant left half are often characterized as analytic and logical, while persons with a dominant right half often may be characterized as imaginative, creative, and emotional. Lateralization is a division of labor rather than a decisive separation. This means that persons dominated by the left half is not without emotion and those dominated by the right is not without the ability to reason logically. This is also because there are many other influences on personal characteristics besides a simple lateral dominance.

12.1.2 The Amygdala

It was about 80 years from Darwin's theory that emotions are related to the brain before Weiskrantz (1956) showed that monkeys lost their natural fear reactions after brain damage. The reactions were similar to reactions observed by Kluver and Bucy in 1939. The damage was localized to the amygdala in both cases. This was the start of the amygdala's reputation as center for emotions in co-operation with several smaller parts which were known as the limbic structures, which is in turn at the center of the early warning system indicated in Sect. 1.8.

Amygdala is a small, almond-shaped structure localized in each of the brain halves at the back of the brain towards the brain stem. It consists of at least a dozen kernels, each with subordinate parts with connections to each other and to other parts of the brain (LeDoux & Phelps, 2008) . Localization of the limbic structure (or system) is indicated both in Figs. 1.4 and 12.1. Figure 12.2 (see page 87) is a close up of the most important parts.

The limbic structure is traditionally localized to the subcortical part of the brain, but results from modern research suggests that localization and dividing lines should not be interpreted as definite. As is argued by Pessoa (2013) localization may be less important than integration in interactions within the brain. It is even after half a Century's research not full agreement on what is part of the limbic structure (Gazzaniga, Ivry, Mangun, & Steven, 2009), and the differentiation of old and new cortex is also less clear after the discovery of structures corresponding to neocortical structures in vertebrates (LeDoux, 2000). There is, notwithstanding, robust evidence that the amygdala is related to emotions. Animals with injuries in the amygdala shows, for instance, generally confused emotional responses and loss of natural fear reactions. Humans with injured amygdala show problems in terms of slow responses to emotional words and difficulties in identifying facial expressions for fear. They also lack fear reactions, but still understand that frightening stimuli may arouse an emotion.

Results from studies have shown that amygdala directs stimulation to a lateral kernel both subcortically and cortically via thalamus. The fear response can be suppressed by an inhibition of this kernel. The two "roads" via thalamus has provided a model for LeDoux's theory that emotions are aroused in two way: By a subcortical, «fast and dirty» road with rough information that there is a problem, and by a slower, cortical road with fine grained information about how the problem might be appraised (LeDoux, 2000; LeDoux & Phelps, 2008). Notice that this might correspond to Lazarus' differentiation of primary and secondary appraisal (see Sect. 6.1.1) Results have, furthermore, shown that information in the lateral kernel is sent to amygdala's basic kernel. The basic kernel seems to function as a central for decisions about reactions, as is indicated by the stop in expression resulting from injuries to this part.

The research on amygdala is an example of the beginning of a map of the brain's role in emotional reactions. This is a map which is continuously corrected. Results from recent studies have, for instance, indicated that amygdala is not decisive for visual detection of stimuli which triggers fear. Pessoa and Adolphs (2010) have referred to the area of the pulvinar nuclei as an alternative. The pulvinar nuclei are localized in the thalamus, have its main connections to the visual cortex, and are central for the attention to relevant stimulation. Visual stimulation with emotional significance has been shown to engage several areas of the brain in addition to the amygdala, i. a. the orbitofrontal cortex, the anterior insula and the anterior cingulate cortex. This suggests that there are several possible inroads which relate to the amygdala as mainly an integrating function (Pessoa & Adolphs, 2010).

Other aspects of the amygdala have been discovered in studies of complex reactions. One example may be that when

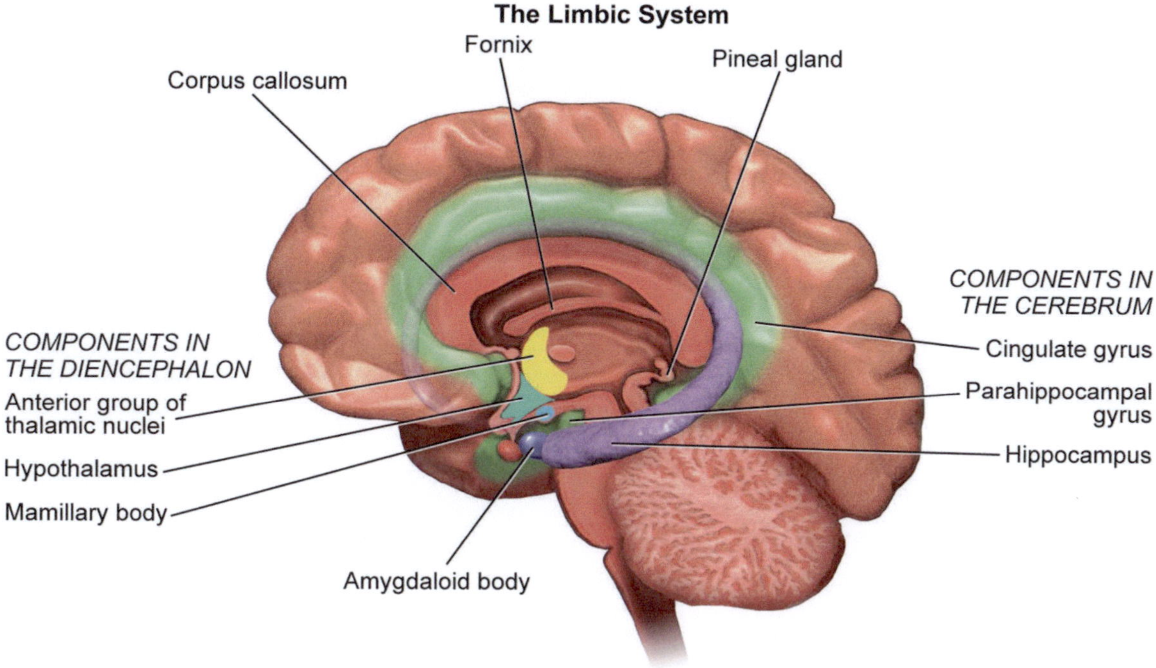

Fig. 12.2 A close up on the limbic system

a rat in a cage learns to fear, for instance a sound, the animal's fear is not only related to the sound but the rat begins to fear the cage as well. The experience of the cage in this way presupposes an ability to remember something. This is managed in the hippocampus, which is the oldest part of the cortex (see Fig. 12.2). The relation of emotions to interaction between the amygdala and the hippocampus is confirmed by tests which show that persons with injuries in the amygdala can predict that a stimulus may lead to fear without actually experiencing the emotion, whereas persons with injury in the hippocampus will show normal fear experiences, but are not able to predict that some fear-arousing stimulus will happen.

A further elaboration of this theme is represented by Olsson and Phelps' (2004, 2007) studies. The authors noted that fear may be learned in three different ways: By direct experience, by observing others' being hurt, for instance by an electric shock, and by being instructed that something is dangerous. They selected 29 students to learn by each of these methods, and used neutral and angry faces on a PC screen as stimuli. The angry faces were presented both unmasked and masked. Students in the direct experience group learnt that angry faces were associated with danger by receiving a mild electric shock when an angry face was shown on the screen. Students in an observation learning group watched a film who showed the reactions of person when an angry face was shown, and students in the instruction group were simply told that angry electric shocks were associated with angry faces on the PC. Emotional arousal was measured by GSR electrodes on two fingers on the left hand. An overview of the set up for the study is shown in Table 12.1 (see page 88).

The results showed no difference in arousal for students in the three groups. Thus, watching the PC screen resulted in about the same GSR reactions for angry faces whether the students had experienced a shock, observed others' response to the face, or being instructed about angry faces. The central result was that reactions on the GSR were shown for masked angry faces only for students in Groups 1 and 2, who received stimulation (angry faces) directly via subcortical connections. This direct connection was not possible for students in Group 3, whose experience of the angry face was dependent on language, i.e. of being instructed about the danger, and, consequently, of cortical connections from the hippocampus.

A stimulation based on the meaning of spoken words is unique for humans, and the results therefore also show that the neurological connections in emotional reactions may be different for animal and man. The demonstration that amygdala responds to linguistic stimulation may, furthermore, mean that arousal of the amygdala may be diminished by talking, i.e. by psychotherapy. This is confirmed in a study which showed that the reappraisal of a scene, for instance of a crying woman, resulted in a diminished reaction in the amygdala (Ochsner, Bunge, Gross, & Gabrielli, 2002). fMRI studies have indicated that this is associated with activation from an area in the left dorsolateral prefrontal cortex (Ochsner et al., 2002; Phelps, 2005).

The overview indicates that the amygdala is an important partner in a network of connections from different part of the brain rather than the very center of emotional reactions. It is also not reserved for emotional processing. Pessoa (2013) cited evidence that amygdala is involved in novelty detection, salience selection and decision making, and shows an integration of functions which is more characteristic of the brain than a mere differentiation of emotion and cognition.

Teil I

Table 12.1 Overview of a test of three types of learning

Set up	Three groups of students were shown neutral, masked and unmasked angry faces on a PC screen. Presentation of angry faces were accompanied with a mild electric shock		
	Group 1	**Group 2**	**Group 3**
Learning	By experience	By observation	By instruction
Response to angry face on screen	Received electric shock	Observed a person receiving electric shock	Were told before-hand that was associated
Measure	Physiological activation measured by GSR		
Result groups 1 and 2		**Result group 3**	
GSM activation both for masked and unmasked angry faces		GSM activation only for unmasked angry faces	

Based on Olsson and Phelps (2007)

12.1.3 Other Emotions

The significance of the studies on the amygdala is limited by being almost exclusively related to one emotion, i.e. fear. The reason for this is, as has been noted by LeDoux (2000), that neuropsychological studies on emotions presuppose unequivocal definitions of both stimulation and emotion. Fear has the large advantage of being easily identified by avoidance- or flight responses which is related to well-known stimuli. Corresponding levels of definitions can be established for disgust, but are very difficult to obtain for other emotions. The large differences between individual emotions which are evident in the descriptions in Chap. 3 suggest that the brain may reserve different areas for different emotions. The need for an integration of cortical information in terms of memory and reflection may, for instance, be much greater for interest and sadness than for surprise and fear.

Differences in neurological background for different emotions are confirmed in a study by Damasio et al. (2000), where participants were instructed to imagine intense, personally experienced episodes of sadness, happiness, anger and fear while their brain activity was registered by PET. The registration started when a GSR measure showed that the persons were beginning to be aroused. The results showed activity both in common- and specific areas. Common activity was registered in insular cortex, secondary somatosensory cortex, cingulate cortex, kernels in the brain stem, tegmentum and the hypothalamus. Specific increased and decreased activity was shown as follows:

Happiness **Increased activity** shown in right part of insula, right secondary somatosensory area (SII), left and right anterior cingulate, right posterior cingulate, right orbitofrontal cortex, left basal forebrain, right hypothalamus and left midbrain.

Decreased activity shown in right prefrontal dorsolateral.

Sadness **Increased activity** shown in ventral and medial prefrontal sector and insula.

Decreased activity shown in right dorsolateral prefrontal cortex, left dorsolateral prefrontal and parietal cortices.

Anger **Increased activity** shown in orbitofrontal and cingulate regions.

Decreased activity shown in bilateral deactivation of SII.

Fear **Increased activity** shown in orbitofrontal and cingulate regions.

Decreased activity shown in lateralized SII.

The list from Damasio et al. (op. cit) can be supplied by Gazzaniga et al.'s (2009) results from studies on the neurological background of anger, sadness, and disgust with fMRI and PET. Anger was associated with the same regions as in Damasio et al. (op. cit.) in results from studies with fMRI and PET from Gazzaniga et al. (2009), who in addition associated fear with the amygdala, sadness with amygdala and the temporal pole, and disgust with insula and the anterior cingulate. Gazzaniga et al. (op. cit.) conceived of the anterior cingulate cortex as a general area for emotions.

Other views on the background of emotions are especially represented by Panksepp's (2004a, b, 2007) studies by the use of electrical and chemical stimulation and PET for the mapping of anatomical and chemical systems in the brain. This has led Panksepp to the conclusion that there are seven systems in the brain which corresponds to instinctive-emotional behaviors (see Sect. 13.5). The seven systems are all assumed to have their background in the brain's grey substance (the periaqueductal grey, PAG). Negative affects (emotions) are found to have a background in dorsal-, and positive affects in ventrale areas of the PAG, with areas for other emotions dispersed between these two. This research, which is supported by Damasio (2010) among others, is somewhat controversial because of the use of a concept of emotion which is unclear to the extent that it is difficult to know what is specifically registered by Panksepp's methods.

It might be noted at the end of this section that large parts of the brain seem to be involved in emotions. Further illustration was contributed by Rosen and Levenson (2009), who reviewed the indications of neurological background related to different phases of emotions, such as sensation and perception, appraisal and experience, regulation of emotions and recognition and understanding of others' emotions. All phases seemed to be connected to several areas, and the areas which seemed to be central to emotions in general were noted as the amygdala, the anterior insula, the parietal lobes, and the dorsolateral, ventrolateral and ventromedial prefrontal cortex.

12.2 Physiological Basis of Emotions

Emotions are influenced by the body's central and peripheral nervous system. Messages from the brain are imparted via chemical substances (transmitter substances, hormones and neuromodulators/peptides) which serve to transmit information at the nerve endings (the synapses). This results in changes which can be measured by several types of measures. Common measures are registrations of changes in the ANS (see Sect. 7.2) with GSR (see Sect. 1.7) and pulse or heart rate (HR, heartbeats pr. minute). A usual set up for this is shown in Fig. 12.3, which also represents the simplest type of a lie detector. Other common measures are EMG (see Sect. 2.6), registration of breathing and eye fixations.

12.2.1 The Central Nervous System

The central nervous system comprises the main part in the body's nervous system. The content I.e. the spinal cord and the brain, have regulating and distributive roles in relation to emotions. Emotional information reaches the skeletal (voluntary) muscles via nerves in the spinal cord. The brain stem at the continuation of the spinal cord comprises the reticular substance with the reticular activation system. This oldest part of the brain is built for regulation of wakefulness and sleep, activation of the body's arousal and preparation of the attention function. This sets a frame for emotional functioning generally, for instance in terms of the rapidity and intensity of emotional activation. The cerebellum, which has its main function in control of the motor apparatus, influences the control and cooperation of emotional impulses by regulating the duration and intensity of emotional expression.

12.2.2 The Peripheral Nervous System

The peripheral nervous system is differentiated into the ANS and the somatic (voluntary) nervous system. The ANS, with its extensive net of nerves, has been by far the largest source of information. Table 7.1 showed the influences on the sympathetic and parasympathetic parts of the ANS, and can be an example that emotions are the key factors for mobilizing energy to meet the challenges in the environment. The model for this was indicated in Sects. 1.2 and 7.4, and comprises a mobilization of energy for adaptive responses, for instance in terms of flight in fear or fight in anger, which includes: (1) Quick breath to deliver more oxygen to the blood. (2) Increase in heartbeats to drive the blood faster to the peripheral parts of

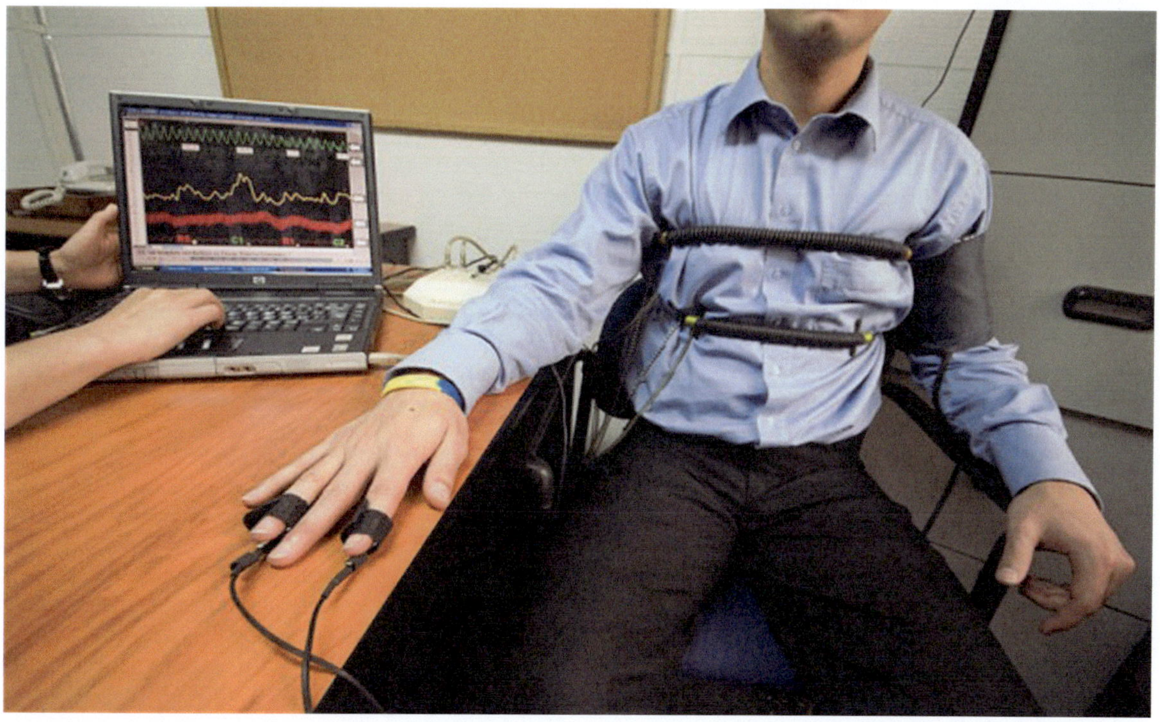

Fig. 12.3 A lie-detector set-up with HR and GSR measures

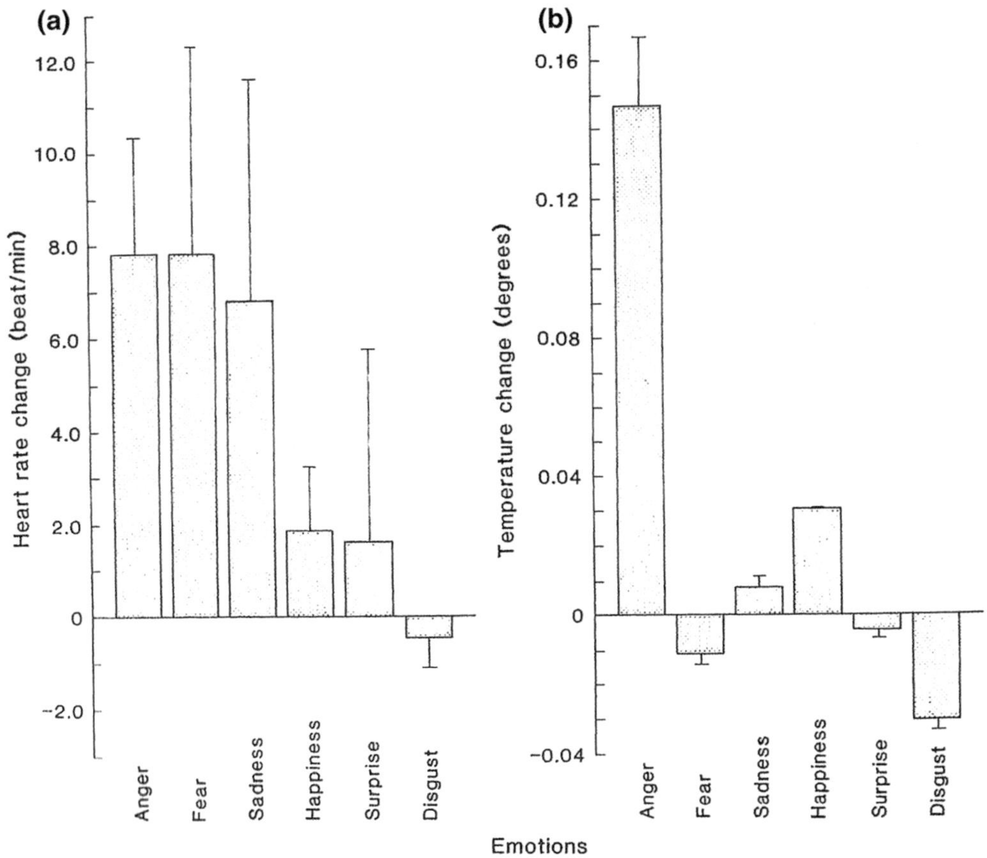

Fig. 12.4 Results from the measurement of HR (**a**) and finger temperature (**b**) for six emotions (from Ekman, Levenson, & Friesen, 1983)

the body. (3) Readiness for action in terms of muscle tension, which resulting in increased sweat on the skin. The changes mean, generally, that energy is directed from the digestive system to an executive organization to prepare the muscles and make the senses more acute. The resulting changes are manifold, and are experienced and interpreted in different ways as was noted in Sect. 4.2. The model may seem more straightforward for negative than for positive emotions. It is, for instance, not self-evident that a linear increase in energy is the best way to support interested examination or play and enjoyment in happiness. These types of behavior may be dependent on parasympathetic stimulation to balance the sympathetic arousal.

There is, as was noted in Sect. 4.2, some indications of experiences associated with ANS reactions related to specific emotions. A question whether there actually are emotion specific responses has far-reaching theoretical significance because it is central to the very concept of differences in emotional types. An example may also be that all the three theories which were cited in Chap. 11 seem to presuppose that such specificity exists. A study designed to answer this question was conducted by Ekman, Levenson, and Friesen (1983), who stimulated participants by imitation of facial expressions and recall of private emotional episodes to arousal of anger, fear, sadness, happiness, surprise, and disgust. Measurement comprised five different indications of ANS responses I.e. HR, GSR in fingers, EMG in the arms and temperatures in the long finger in both hands, and was conducted from the start of the arousal and until it ended. Examples of results from the study are shown in Fig. 12.4, which shows HR and finger temperatures.

The results shown in Fig. 12.4 shows that there were some differences related to the individual indices, for instance in HR for anger, fear, and sadness, but that they were not impressive. The authors argued however that the variation related to emotion type was expected and shown for the combination, or response pattern, on the different measures. Such variation may be suggested by the differences in finger temperatures for the three emotions.

Ekman et al.'s (1983) study has both been criticized and supported by later studies. A thorough review of studies by Cacioppo and co-workers (Larsen, Berntson, Poehlmann, Ito, & Cacioppo, 2008) showed that there are some indications of ANS-reactions associated with specific emotions. Anger, fear, and sadness seem, for instance to be related to higher HR increase than disgust, anger has been related to higher blood pressure than fear, and disgust seems to relate to greater GSR increase than fear. It has also been shown, as was indicated in Chap. 7, that anger are more closely associated with cardiovascular problems than fear. The conclusion of a more recent review has been that there are robust differences in ANS-activation of positive and negative emotions, but that differences within each of these categories are small and unclear (Mauss & Robinson, 2009).

These examples shows little background for a proposal that there are emotion specific activations of the ANS. Results are, on the other hand, not sufficient to refute a proposal about specific activation. The question is not answered by reference to convincing evidence because it is extremely difficult to obtain simultaneous measures from a large set of instruments at comparable levels of intensity of emotions. If intensity levels are not constant it is not possible to separate effects of intensity and effects of emotion type, e.g. effects of a high intensity of anger and a mild intensity of fear. Unfortunately, a control for intensity level of arousal was not included in Ekman et al.'s (1983), or in most other studies of emotion specificity.

12.3 Neurochemical Influences on Emotions

Part of the causal chain is that chemical transmission of information at the nerve endings are transported further to an arousal of emotions. This means that emotions are influenced by biochemical reactions, especially in the form of neurotransmitters and hormones. Examples of chemical influence mentioned in the descriptions of ANS and the HPA-axis (see Sect. 7.2) was adrenalin and cortisol. The chemical factors which seem to be associated with emotional reactions are testosterone and noradrenaline in anger, serotonin in fear/anxiety, dopamine in interest, oxytocin and prolactin in sadness, and oxytocin and opioids in happiness (Panksepp & Biven, 2012).

There is a large practical potential related to chemical influences. This is long since recognized by pharmaceutical firms who have developed medicines who may inhibit experiences of sadness and anxiety. Chemical influences have also been known and used for thousands of years in different parts of the world. Examples are chewing of coca leaves in South America and Khat in Eastern Africa for their calming effects, and the use of hashish in Northern Africa and opium in Asia to obtain positive emotions. The trend in recent times has been to develop synthetic chemical stimulations with strong dependency effects aimed at the stimulation of intense and positive emotional experiences.

12.4 Summary

The background for emotional reactions in the body are studied within anatomy and neurology, which try to identify the areas of the brain which are associated with emotional reactions, and within physiology, which is aimed at discovering the effect of emotional arousal on the functioning of the body.

Emotional reactions are lateralized to the right hemisphere in the brain.

Many studies have confirmed that the almond-shaped amygdala downwards at the back of the brain is involved both in fear which is triggered subcortically and fear reactions based on memory by connection to the hippocampus.

There is further evidence of specific localization of happiness, sadness, anger, and disgust. Areas which seem to be generally involved in emotional reactions are the orbitofrontal and cingulate cortex and insula. The frame for emotional activation is set by the reticular system on top of the spinal cord. The reticular system regulates the basic functions of the body.

Physiological responses associated with emotions are most directly related to the sympathetic part of the ANS. The main chain of reactions is from an redirection of energy from digestion to the mobilization of the senses and the motor apparatus. Studies on emotion specific activation in the ANS have provided evidence of a differentiation in the activation of positive and negative emotions, but there is a lack of conclusive evidence in relation to differences within these types. There are, however, indications that anger, fear, and sadness are associated with larger increase in heart rate than disgust, and that anger is related to higher blood pressure than fear and that disgust results in larger skin conductance than fear.

It is well known that emotions are influenced by chemical means. Examples are medicines for depression and anxiety and several types of intoxicants.

Reflection Questions

1. Much of our knowledge of the biological bases of emotions has been contributed by animal research. What are the advantages and limitations of this research for the understanding of emotions in humans?
2. The amygdala is traditionally conceived as a localized hub of emotional stimulation. This seems recently to be challenged by a concept of amygdala as an integrating part in a neural network. What different implications can follow from these viewpoints as regards the role of experience in the formation of the biological basis of emotions, and how do each of them relate to the concept of the brain as a dynamic system?

Research/Exercise Examples

1 The results from Damasio et al.'s (2000) study (see Sect. 12.1.3) indicated that emotions may alter the brain. Which other examples can you mention? The same results also showed that emotions were results of cognition, and that cognition consequently may alter the brain. But is not both cognition and emotion already in the brain? Discuss the implication of this by reference to the anatomy of the brain.

2 Even with access to the best fMRI and PET scanning techniques you would still have problems in investigating emotion-related brain activity because the activity must be related to an emotion. How would you make a set-up to secure that the activity in the brain referred to a specific emotion?

Further Reading

Damasio, A. R. (1994). *Descartes' error. Emotion, reason and the human brain*. New York: Putnam.

Gazzaniga, M. S., Ivry, R. B., & Mangun, G. R. (2013). *Cognitive neuroscience. The biology of the mind.* (4th ed.). New York: Norton.

Pessoa, L. (2013). *The cognitive-emotional brain. From interactions to integration*. Cambridge, MA: The MIT Press.

Final Remarks

13

This chapter starts with some limitation of the book and criticism of the book's "modal" viewpoint that emotions are (a) activated automatically when something in registered by the senses and (b) show an integrated response of several components. It is recognized that the evidence-based knowledge cited in the book refers to a simplified version of reality. Emotions in this "scientific" reality are experienced one at a time as short responses, which is in contrast to the frequent blending and long-time duration of "real life" emotions. The text is, accordingly, supplied with short notes on blending and long-time duration of emotions.

This chapter is closed with a discussion on animals' emotion. It is noted that animals possess the limbic system which seem to play a major part in basic emotions. Some animals (gorillas, chimpanzees, orangutans, and dolphins) have even been shown to pass the test of self-consciousness, and may be assumed to have some self-conscious emotions. There is, notwithstanding, still an open question whether animals possess the cognitive development that is required for the ordinary emotions which are developed around the child's first birthday.

13.1 General View

The aim of this book has been to describe the main concepts, basic approaches and areas in the study of emotions. It has been necessary to shorten almost all subjects and themes to the bone. This has resulted in the loss of quite some nuances, and of many alternative interpretations. The presentation may, therefore, at times seem superficial and rigid and citing "truths" that are not sufficiently founded in evidence. It is, therefore, important to note that all areas in the study of emotions are dynamic. They are full of questions which are not adequately answered and therefore in need of further exploration. Thus, the book is by no means a complete report on the subject of emotions. It may, hopefully, be the start of a beginning with literature references to those who seek further information.

Several areas have either not been conceived as central to insight into emotions as defined in the present book, or have been left out because of not pertaining to research on emotions' basic, general characteristics. Foremost among the left out areas are sociological (e.g. Turner, 2009) and anthropological (e.g. Beatty, 2013) research, and psychiatric and psychological studies of emotional disorders. Also left out is a large literature on applied work with emotions, mainly psychotherapy (Greenberg, 2011), approaches to stimulate understanding of emotions in children (Gottman & Declaire, 1997), and emotional intelligence in leaders and other personnel in the workplace (Goleman, 1998).

Emotions are generally conceived of as something «warm» and «dynamic» which is easily moved, and which is associated with suffering and ecstasy, attraction, rage, black sadness and with a happiness which is felt as an uplifting of the whole body. But this is the poets', the singers', and at times the painters' world. They all try to articulate the emotions' varied experiences, expressions and uniqueness. Scientific work may, by comparison, seem slow, rigid, and unimaginative. This is because science is aimed at the discovery of general laws which may influence the living of our life. Interesting and individual variations are useless distractions and noise in this context. The difference is, however, not definite because emotions refer to phenomena that are intensely personal, i.e. which exist in individual persons' experience and body. That is, in a majority point of view, there are also recent viewpoints that emotions are phenomena which circulates not only in social life (Ahmed, 2004), but may also be part of nature (Massumi, 2002; Thrift, 2008; see Wetherell, 2012).

The content of the book is comprised by a consensus about emotions which has been referred to as a "modal" viewpoint. This is a viewpoint where emotions are conceived as activated automatically when something in the surroundings is registered by the senses. An argument against the modal concept is that emotional experience is not just a result of sensations, but is also part of- and contributes to determine what is being sensed. An example may be that a person does not respond as automatically to a negative behavior from a close friend as from a negative behavior from a stranger (Feldman Barrett, Ochsner & Gross, 2007).

A. Vikan, *A Fast Road to the Study of Emotions*,
DOI 10.1007/978-3-319-52313-2_13

Another argument against the modal concept is that the word "emotions" is a generalization or a «box» with heterogeneous objects. Lay persons' and experts' word "fear" is, for instance, taken to refer to a variation of behaviors from fleeing from an angry dog to crossing fingers or shifting visual fixation in order to contain a mild anxiety in a group meeting. This alternative view is central to Russell and Feldman Barrett's theory (see Sect. 11.4.2), and may open new doors for the understanding of emotions. But this is still not an alternative which is supported by sufficient research. It cannot serve as a reinterpretation of the diverse emotional phenomena which have been described in this book.

There is some support for «anti-modal» arguments in results from studies which is related to the modal assumption that emotion can be defined as a composite of three types of components (see Fig. 1.2). Bradley and Lang (2000) pointed out that studies have not proven that there is in fact a close association of the components. The co-variations between measures of self-ratings, behavior, and physiological reactions in a well-defined emotion such as fear have, for instance, only explained a small part (10–15%) of the total variation. Bradley and Lang's (2000) argument cannot be regarded as decisive because there is no evident basis for equivalence in measures of the different types of components. The ordinal points of the rating scales which employed in measures of experience are, for instance, far from being equivalent to the interval scales of GSR measures of physiological responses.

The content of the book is based on what can be learnt from systematic studies. Systematic research can only be conducted in relation to specific aspects of a phenomenon. They are, thus, focused on a simplified version of the very reality that they are designed to discover. The simplified version of emotions in this book is that there are different types of emotions which are experienced one at a time at relatively low intensities. These emotions are held to represent a well-defined, short response to a specific causal stimulus or event in the surrounding or in a person's perceptions, memories, or thoughts. Real emotions, by contrast, are often experienced as a blended emotional reaction which can vary in intensity from very mild to absorbing and frightening intense, and which may be repeated and last over years in relation to unclear causes. There has been some reference both to intensity (see Sects. 2.2 and 4.3) and blending (see Sects. 3.4 and 7.1), but duration has been left out of the discussion.

13.2 Emotional Blending

Emotional blending means that a person experiences two or more simultaneous emotions for another person, an event or an object. The most usual blending is simultaneous experiences of fear and interest and fear and anger. Sadness and anger, sadness and shame, and surprise and happiness are also frequent combinations. It is not unusual that more than two emotions are blended. Surprise, disgust and fear may, for instance, be blended into strong dislike reactions to something, while anger, sadness and guilt are often represented in the same negative reaction to other persons. There has been no follow up on Izard's (1972) early studies which indicated that both anxiety and depression may be composed of both negative and positive emotions, and there is, consequently, very little research on this subject.

Blending was noted as a problem in Sect. 3.4, and it was proposed that this might relate to the experience of two different emotions for the same object or event. A further examination may reveal that blending pertains to a simultaneous experience of different aspects of a causal agent. Perception of a lion in a cage leads generally to a fear of the dangerous animal, and is blended very quickly by feelings of interest when one realizes that the animal is harmless. But the fear is still present as the cage is approached for a close inspection the animal. The can be proposed that the blending in this case is maintained by quick shifts in experiences and memories into the experience of an emotionally blended conscious stream.

Blending may result in problems both because of the links between emotions and behavior (see Sect. 1.2) and because of self-understanding. The links between emotions and behavior means that the different emotions in a blending are experienced as tendencies of different behaviors or "action tendencies" (see Sect. 8.4). Action tendencies in the lion example are to flee because of the fear and to approach because of the interest. These behaviors are mutually exclusive, and a probable result is that the person is paralyzed, i.e. the emotions do not function to support the person's adaption to the situation.

Blending comprise a problem to self-understanding because this is dependent on clearly differentiated alternatives and aims at clear and definitive conclusions. This means that a person seeks to define him/herself as competent at something, preferring something and avoiding something. A blending in this context does not provide an alternative because a person cannot define her-himself as somebody who is part or percent of one or the other. The problems are most evident in relationships to the closest persons, who provoke both the strongest positive and negative emotions. Frequent blended experiences of, for instance, happiness and anger, lead to doubt whether one «actually» loves or hates the other followed by confusion as to what kind of person may have such mixed emotions, and further to testing of this by a mix of behaviors which leads to new emotions of sadness and guilt, to new blends and to new confusion etc. This comprises imbalances and conflicts both between persons and inside individuals which has often served as dramatic themes in novels and plays.

13.3 Duration of Emotions

It is a general experience that emotions last much longer than the moment in which they are aroused. An explanation of this must comprise the variation from a few minutes in Mary's reactions to months and years in Silvia's continuous emotional preoccupation in Fig. 1.1. The long duration of emotions is often used as an argument against the theory that emotions consist of neural circuits. A variant of this argument is that emotions which are aroused by examination marks and country music, such as John and Silvia's emotions in Fig. 1.1 are results of many years of development and learning. They cannot, therefore, be part of neurological circuits which were evolved millions of years ago. Another argument is that emotions cannot support and be part of adaption if they do not continue to help mobilize energy e.g. until a flight or a fight has succeeded. A third argument is that emotions are not only present during some adaptive task. They also pop up when the person has nothing to do and where there is no obvious adaptive challenge.

The reason for these critical viewpoints on «circuit theory» is that emotions seem to be tied to memories, and therefore to cognition. Chapter 6 comprised two further examples of this. The first is the flashbulb memories and studies of the effect of emotional intensity which suggested that emotions «stamp» the memory for significant experiences. These «stamped» memories are shown in emotionally arousing flashbacks which are symptoms and major problems in patients diagnosed with post-traumatic disorder (PTSD). The second example is that the congruence principle suggests that emotions is integrated into both memory and thinking. It was suggested than happiness stimulates a congruence which instigates, opens or releases the memory of other positive stimuli and events which reinforces happiness and leads to further congruence, and so on.

Both examples suggest that emotion and cognition are so closely associated that they are aspects of the same psychological processes rather than being separate and differentiated parts. This is supported by a review of neuroscience research which suggested that information from the senses and the appraisal of this information are parts of the same brain system (Duncan & Feldman Barrett, 2007)S. The authors argued that this pertains to information which is necessary and mutually dependent in the adaption, and which comprise the neurological representation of cognition and emotion. The duration of the emotions can be conceived as an example of this two-part process. The differentiation of emotion and cognition by ordinary persons as well as emotion scientists may, consequently, refer to their *experience* of a difference rather than to a *real* difference between processes.

13.4 Do We Always Have Emotions?

A question about duration and the connection of emotions and cognition leads naturally to a question whether we always have emotions. The answer to the question is "yes" based on the viewpoint that an emotion is a signal that something is important to the organism. Emotions refer in this respect to an arousal of energy which is necessary and sufficient to mobilize an experience. This is parallel to Izard's (2009) and Frijda's (2007) suggestion that interest is a primary emotion which provokes the consciousness to be linked to the surrounding and provide the point of departure for all other emotions.

These viewpoints mean that consciousness implies emotions, and that we are, consequently, always "emotional" in so far as we are awake. An argument to the contrary may be that consciousness presupposes intentionality, and that we are not always goal-oriented in our everyday experience. We may, for instance, swing to and forth and be without plans or directions, and therefore be without emotions over some time. Another argument is that consciousness and behavior is mobilized by needs like hunger and thirst, which are outside of the definition of emotions. We should not, therefore, assume that we are always feeling some emotions, but the question is both necessary and useful in order to reflect on the degree to which our lives are filled with emotions.

13.5 Do Animals Have Emotions?

This book has been limited to emotions in humans, but examples of emotional expressions in animals were shown in Fig. 2.2, and results from many studies cited in Chap. 12 were conducted on animals. The examples suggest that there is agreement among experts that animals have emotions. This is supported by, as was referred to in 12.1, that emotions are anatomically based on the subcortical limbic system, which is very similar in animals and humans. The chemical and hormonal processes in the body are also very similar. Mammals are, for instance, rapidly dependent on the same narcotic substances as humans. The main question in this respect is probably how to demarcate what is meant by emotions. Should emotions, for instance, be extended to insects, as was done by Darwin (see 1.5), and to snakes, as is indicated by anecdotal evidence by Bekoff (2007)?

Humans have, on the other hand, a unique position due to the development of the neocortex, which enables extended memory, abstract thinking and reasoning and a large reinforcement of the usefulness of these new functions by the development of language capabilities. The new functions in the neocortex makes possible a complex and coherent emotional life where each emotion can be extended by thoughts and memories related to the experience (Hart, 2009). These are the main reasons why humans, in contrast to animals, are able to hide their emotions and act as if they have other emotions than their actual ones by, for instance, smile and seem happy when they are actually angry or sad. Humans are also, in contrast to animals, able to regulate their emotions in various ways and to refer to emotions with words and to talk about them after they have happened. To name just some basic differences.

The examples may suggest that animals and humans may have the basic emotional reactions in common, and that the experience component in humans comprise a much larger degree of consciousness, coherence and control. This may mean that basic emotions are similar, and that animals do not have neurological support for a cognitive development which results in ordinary emotions when the human child is about one year old. This leads to an assumption that animals do not obtain the necessary cognitive development for the self-conscious emotions shame, guilt, pride, envy, and jealousy.

Results from studies warn against very strong conclusions in this area. Apes most similar to humans (gorilla, chimpanzee and orangutan) and dolphins have been shown to pass the classical test for self-consciousness (Denton, 2009). The test consists of marking a child, an ape or a dolphin without their awareness on a visible part (e.g. the face) by a distinct mark (e.g. a red point) which they can only perceive in a mirror. A child reacts typically from about their 18th month by trying to remove the mark on their face after having tried to remove the mark from the mirror when they were younger (Amsterdam, 1972). Apes' and dolphins' reactions are likewise directed at their own body and not at the mirror. The interpretation of this behavior is that it shows a realization on part of these subjects that they understand that the mirror is mirroring themselves, which presuppose some concept that they are a "self", or something similar, which is being shown in the mirror.

The large problem for comparative studies is, of course, that animals are not able to tell about their emotion experiences. The must be "asked" in terms of behavioral tasks. Panksepp and Biven (2012) reported, as was mentioned in 12.1, that they had been able to identify seven types of behavior which corresponded to seven emotions in terms of instinctive-emotional behavioral patterns common to animals and humans. The seven patterns were: Seeking (interest), fear/anxiety, rage/anger, desire (sexual excitement), concern (love and attachment), panic/grief (sadness) and play/happiness. This corresponds, except for desire and concern, to most list of basic emotions. The patterns are proposed in the Darwinian sense as fundamental characteristics of an evolutionary process where there is no dividing line between animals and humans.

Reflection Questions

1. What can you know about a person in some context when you identify her/his emotion?
2. How would you differentiate emotions from needs such as hunger, thirst, sex and sleep?

Research/Exercise Examples

1. Which are the main characteristics of human emotions? (You should be able to answer this question with a very few sentences after reading this book).
2. You may have a funding of $10 million if you can design a project that will result in a new and better understanding of human emotions. What will be your priorities, and why?

Further Reading

Hermans, D., Rime, B., & Mesquita, B. (2013). *Changing emotion*. New York: Psychology Press.

Panksepp, J., & Biven, L. (2012). *The archaeology of mind*. New York: Norton.

Wetherell, M. (2012). *Affect and emotion*. London: Sage.

References

Abraham, R. (2005). Emotional intelligence in the workplace: A review and synthesis. In R. Schulze & R. D. Roberts (Eds.), *Emotional intelligence* (pp. 255–270). Cambridge, Massachusetts: Hogrefe & Hogrefe.

Abu-Lughod, L. (1986). *Veiled sentiments*. Berkeley: University of California Press.

Ackerman, B. P., Abe, J. A., & Izard, C. E. (1998). Differential emotions theory and emotional development: Mindful of modularity. In M. F. Mascolo & S. Griffin (Eds.), *What develops in emotional development?* (pp. 85–106). New York: Plenum Press.

Ahmed, S. (2004). *The cultural politics of emotion*. New York: Routledge.

Aldwin, C. M. (1994). *Stress, coping, and development*. New York: Guilford.

Alexander, F. (1939). Psychological aspects of medicine. *Psychosomatic Medicine, 1,* 7–18.

Alexander, F. (1950). *Psychosomatic medicine: It's principles and applications*. New York: Norton.

American Psychiatric Association. (2013). *Diagnostic and statistics manual of mental disorders* (5th ed.). Washington, DC: APA.

Amsterdam, B. (1972). Mirror self-object reactions before age two. *Developmental Psychobiology, 5,* 297–305.

Anisman, H. (2014). *Introduction to stress and health*. New York: Sage.

Aristotle. (2000). Nicomachean ethics (translated by Roger Crisp) Cambridge: Cambridge University Press.

Arnold, M. B. (1968). *The nature of emotion: Selected readings*. Harmondsworth: Penguin.

Ashforth, B. E., & Humphrey, R. H. (1995). Emotion in the workplace: A reappraisal. *Human Relations, 48,* 97–125.

Austin, E. J., Saklofske, D. H., & Egan, V. (2005). Personality, well-being and health correlates of trait emotional intelligence. *Personality and Individual Differences, 38,* 547–558.

Banerjee, M. (1997). Peeling the onion: A multilayered view of children's emotional development. In S. Hala (Ed.), *The development of social cognition* (pp. 241–272). East Sussex: Psychology Press.

Bar-On, R. (1997). *The Bar-On emotional quotient inventory (EQ-I): Technical manual*. Toronto, Canada: Multi-Health Systems.

Bar-On, R. (2000). Emotional and social intelligence: Insights from the emotional quotient inventory. In R. Bar-On & J. D. A. Parker (Eds.), *Handbook of emotional intelligence: Theory, development, assessment, and application at home, school, and in the workplace* (pp. 363–388). San Fransisco: Jossey-Bass.

Barbuto, J. E., Gottfredson, R. K., & Searle, T. P. (2014). An examination of emotional intelligence as an antecedent of servant leadership. *Journal of Leadership and Organizational Studies, 21,* 315–323.

Bargh, J. A., & Williams, J. E. (2007). The nonconscious regulation of emotion. In J. J. Gross (Ed.), *Handbook of emotion regulation* (pp. 429–445). New York: The Guilford Press.

Baron-Cohen, S. (1995). *Mindblindness*. Cambridge, Massachusetts: MIT Press.

Baron-Cohen, S. (1995). *Mindblindness: An essay on autism and theory of mind*. Cambridge, MA: MIT Press.

Barsade, S. (2002). The ripple effect: Emotional contagion and its influence on group behavior. *Administrative Science Quarterly, 47,* 644–675.

Bartlett, E. S., & Izard, C. E. (1972). A dimensional and discrete emotions investigation of the subjective experience of emotion. In C. E. Izard (Ed.), *Patterns of emotion: A new analysis of anxiety and depression* (pp. 129–175). New York: Academic Press.

Beatty, A. (2013). Current emotion research in anthropology: Reporting the field. *Emotion Review, 5,* 414–422.

Bekoff, M. (2007). *The emotional life of animals*. Novato, California: New World Library.

Benedict, R. (1946). *The chrysanthemum and the sword*. Oxford, UK: Houghton Mifflin.

Biron, M., & van Veldhoven, M. (2012). Emotional labour in service work: psychological flexibility and emotion regulation. *Human Relations, 65,* 1259–1282.

Blanchette, I., & Richards, A. (2010). The influence of affect on higher level cognition: a review of research on interpretation, judgment, decision making and reasoning. *Cognition and Emotion, 24,* 561–595.

Blanchflower, D. G. (2009). International evidence on well-being. In A. B. Krueger (Ed.), *Measuring the subjective well-being of nations* (pp. 155–226). Chicago: The University of Chicago Press.

Borke, H., & Su, S. (1972). Perception of emotional responses to social interactions by Chinese and American children. *Journal of Cross-Cultural Psychology, 3,* 309–314.

Bower, G. H. (1981). Mood and memory. *American Psychologist, 36,* 129–148.

Boyatzis, R. E., & Sala, F. (2004). The emotional competence inventory (ECI). In G. Geher (Ed.), *Measuring emotional intelligence: Common ground and controversy* (pp. 143–178). Hauppauge, NY: Nova Science Publishing.

Bradley, M. M., & Lang, P. J. (2000). Measuring emotion; behavior, feeling, and Physiology. In R. D. Lane & L. Nadel (Eds.), *Cognitive neuroscience of emotion* (pp. 242–276). Oxford UK: Oxford University Press.

Bretherton, I., McNew, S., & Beeghly-Smith, M. (1981). Early person knowledge as expressed in gestural, and verbal communication: When do infants acquire a theory of mind? In M. Lamb & L. R. Sherrod (Eds.), *Infant social Cognition* (pp. 333–374). Hillsdale, New Jersey: Erlbaum.

Breugelmans, S. M., Poortinga, Y. H., Ambadazar, Z., Setiadi, B., Vaca, J. B., Widiyanto, P., et al. (2005). Body sensations associated with emotions in Raramuri Indians, rural Javanese, and three student samples. *Emotion, 5,* 166–174.

Briggs, J. L. (1970). *Never in anger. Portrait of an Eskimo family*. Cambridge, MA: Harvard University Press.

Briner, R. B. (1999). The neglect and importance of emotions at work. *European Journal of Work and Organizational Psychology, 8,* 323–346.

A. Vikan, *A Fast Road to the Study of Emotions*,
https://doi.org/10.1007/978-3-319-52313-2

Bringle, R. G. (1991). Psychosocial aspects of jealousy: A transactional model. In P. Salovey (Ed.), *The psychology of jealousy and envy* (pp. 103–131). New York: Guilford.

Brody, L. R. (2000). The socialization of gender differences in emotion expression: Display rules, infant temperament, and differentiation. In A. H. Fischer (Ed.), *Gender and emotion* (pp. 24–47). Cambridge, UK: Cambridge University Press.

Brotheridge, C. M., & Grandey, A. A. (2002). Emotional labor and burnout: Comparing two perspectives of "People work". *Journal of Vocational Behavior, 60,* 17–39.

Brotheridge, C. M., & Lee, R. T. (2003). Development and validation of the Emotional Labor Scale. *Journal of Occupational and Organizational Psychology, 76,* 365–379.

Bull-Schaefer, R. A., & Palanski, M. E. (2013). Emotional contagion at work: An in-class experiential activity. *Journal of Management Education, 38,* 533–559.

Bush, L., Barr, C., McHugo, G., & Lanzetta, J. (1989). The effects of facial control and facial mimicry on subjective reactions to comedy routines. *Motivation and Emotion, 13,* 31–52.

Bushman, B. J. (1995). Moderating role of trait aggressiveness in the effects of violent media on aggression. *Journal of Personality and Social Psychology, 69,* 950–960.

Byrne, D. (1961). The repression-sensitization scale: Rationale, reliability and validity. *Journal of Personality, 29,* 334–349.

Cannon, W. B. (1927). The James-Lange theory of emotions: A critical examination and an alternative. *American Journal of Psychology, 39,* 106–124.

Cannon, W. B. (1927). The James-Lange theory of emotions: a critical examination and an alternative. *American Journal of Psychology, 39,* 106–124.

Caruso, D. R., Bienn, B., & Kornacki, S. A. (2006). Emotional intelligence in the workplace. In J. Ciarrochi, J. P. Forgas, & J. D. Mayer (Eds.), *Emotional Intelligence in everyday life* (pp. 187–205). New York: Psychology Press.

Christianson, S.-Å. (1994). *Traumatiska minnen (Traumatic memories)*. Stockholm: Natur och Kultur.

Clark, D. M. (1999). Anxiety disorders: why they persist and how to treat them. *Behaviour Research and Therapy, 37,* 5–27.

Clark, C. A., & Beck, A. T. (1999). *Scientific foundations of cognitive theory and therapy of depression*. New York: Wiley.

Coan, J. A., & Allen, J. J. B. (Eds.). (2007). *Handbook of emotion elicitation and assessment*. Oxford, UK: Oxford University Press.

Coyne, J. C. (1976). Depression and the response to others. *Journal of Abnormal Psychology, 85,* 186–193.

Crego, A., Martinez-Inigo, D., & Tschan, F. (2013). Moderate effects of attributions on the relationship between emotional dissonance and surface acting: A transactional approach to health care professionals' emotion work. *Journal of Applied Social Psychology, 43,* 570–581.

Damasio, A. R. (1999). *The feeling of what happens: Body and emotion in the making of consciousness*. New York: Harcourt Brace.

Damasio, A. (2010). *Self comes to mind*. London: Heinemann.

Damasio, A. R., Grabowski, T. J., Bechara, A., Damasio, H., Ponto, L. L. B., Parvizi, J., et al. (2000). Subcortical and cortical activity during the feeling of self-generated emotions. *Nature Neuroscience, 3,* 1049–1056.

Damasio, A. R. (1994). Descartes' error. *Emotion, reason and the human brain*. New York: Putnam.

Damasio, A. R. (1994). Descartes' error. *Emotion, reason and the human brain*. New York: Putnam.

Darwin, C. (1872). *The expression of the emotions in man and animals*. London: Albemarle.

Darwin, C. (1872). *The expression of the emotions in man and animals*. London: Albemarle.

Decety, J. (2010). To what extent is the experience of empathy mediated by shared neural circuits? *Emotion Review, 2,* 204–207.

Denton, D. (2009). *The primordial emotions*. Oxford: University Press.

Derryberry, D., & Rothbart, M. K. (1997). Reactive and effortful processes in the organization of temperament. *Developmental Psychopathology, 9,* 633–652.

Diamond, J. (2012). *The world until yesterday*. Ney York: Viking.

Dias, M., Vikan, A., & Gravås, S. (2000). Tentativa de criancas em lidar com as emocoes de raiva e tristeza (Children's regulation of anger and sadness). *Estudos de Psicologia, 5,* 49–70.

Dimberg, U., Thunberg, M., & Elmehed, K. (2000). Unconscious facial reactions to emotional facial expressions. *Psychological Science, 11,* 86–89.

Dimberg, U., Thunberg, M., & Elmehed, K. (2000). Unconscious facial reactions to emotional facial expressions. *Psychological Science, 11,* 86–89.

Doherty, R. W. (1997). The emotional contagion scale: A measure of individual differences. *Journal of Nonverbal Behavior, 21,* 131–154.

Duclos, S. E., Laird, J. D., Schneider, E., Sexter, M., Stern, L., & van Lighten, O. (1989). Emotion specific effects of facial expressions and postures on emotional experience. *Journal of Social and Personality Psychology, 57,* 100–108.

Duncan, S., & Feldman Barrett, L. (2007). Affect is a form of cognition: A neurobiological analysis. *Cognition and Emotion, 21,* 1184–1211.

Dunn, J. (1994). Experience and understanding of emotions, relationships, and membership in a particular culture. In P. Ekman & R. J. Davidson (Eds.), *The nature of emotion. Fundamental questions* (pp. 352–355). Oxford: Oxford University Press.

Earley, P. C., & Gibson, C. B. (1998). Taking stock in our progress on collectivism-individualism: 100 years of solidarity and community. *Journal of Management, 24,* 224–265.

Eibl-Eibesfeldt, I. (1973). The expressive behavior of the deaf-and-blind-born. In M. von Cranach & I. Vine (Eds.), *Social communication and movement* (pp. 163–194). London: Academic Press.

Ekman, P. (1972). Universals and cultural differences in facial expressions of emotion. In J. Cole (Ed.), *Nebraska Symposium on Motivation, 1971* (pp. 207–283). Lincoln: University of Nebraska Press.

Ekman, P. (1994). All emotions are basic. In P. Ekman & R. J. Davidson (Eds.), *The nature of emotion* (pp. 15–19). New York: Oxford University Press.

Ekman, P., & Friesen, W. (1975). *Unmasking the human face: A guide to recognizing emotions from facial expressions*. Englewood Cliffs, NJ: Prentice-Hall.

Ekman, P., Friesen, W. V., & Ellsworth, P. (1972). *Emotion in the human face*. New York: Pergamon Press.

Ekman, P., Levenson, R. W., & Friesen, W. V. (1983). Autonomic nervous system activity distinguishes among emotions. *Science, 221,* 1208–1210.

Ekman, P. (1973). Cross-cultural studies of facial expression. In I P. Ekman (Ed.), *Darwin and facial expression* (pp. 169–222). New York: Academic Press.

Ekman, P. (1973). Cross-cultural studies of facial expression. In P. Ekman (Ed.), *Darwin and facial expression* (pp. 169–222). New York: Academic Press.

Elias, N. (2000). *The civilizing process*. Oxford, UK: Blackwell.

Ellsworth, P. C., & Smith, C. A. (1988). From appraisal to emotion: differences among unpleasant feelings. *Motivation and Emotion, 12,* 271–302.

Endler, N. S., & Kocovski, N. L. (2001). State and trait anxiety revisited. *Journal of Anxiety Disorders, 15,* 231–245.

Endler, N. S., & Parker, J. D. A. (1994). Assessment of multidimensional coping: Task, emotion and avoidance strategies. *Psychological Assessment, 1994*(6), 50–60.

Enticott, P. G., Johnston, P. J., Herring, S. E., Koy, K. E., & Fitzgerald, P. B. (2008). Mirror neuron activation is associated with facial emotion processing. *Neuropsychologica, 46,* 2851–2854.

Feldman Barrett, L. (2006). Are emotions natural kinds? *Perspectives on Psychological Science, 1,* 28–58.

Feldman Barrett, L. F. (2005). Feeling is perceiving: Core affect and conceptualization in the experience of emotion. In L. F. Barrett, P. M. Niedenthal, & P. Winkielman (Eds.), *Emotion and consciousness* (pp. 255–286). New York: The Guilford Press.

Feldman Barrett, L., Ochsner, K. N., & Gross, J. J. (2007). On the automaticity of emotion. In J. A. Bargh (Ed.), *Social psychology and the unconscious* (pp. 173–218). New York: Psychology Press.

Feldman Barrett, L., & Russell, J. A. (1998). Independence and bipolarity in the structure of current affect. *Journal of Personality and Social Psychology, 4,* 967–984.

Finkenauer, C., & Rime, B. (1998). Keeping emotional memories secret: Health and subjective well-being when emotions are not shared. *Journal of Health Psychology, 3,* 47–58.

Finucane, M. L., Alhakami, A., Slovic, P., & Johnson, S. M. (2000). The affect heuristics in judgments of risks and benefits. *Journal of Behavioral Decision Making, 13,* 1–17.

Fischer, A. H. (1993). Sex differences in emotionality: Fact or stereotype? *Feminism and Psychology, 3,* 303–318.

Fischer, A. H., & Manstead, A. S. R. (2000). The relation between gender and emotion in different cultures. In A. H. Fischer (Ed.), *Gender and emotion* (pp. 71–97). Cambridge, UK: Cambridge University Press.

Folkman, S., & Lazarus, R. S. (1980). An analysis of coping in a middle-aged community sample. *Journal of Health and Social Behavior, 21,* 219–239.

Forgas, J. P., & Moylan, S. J. (1987). After the movies: the effects of transient mood states on social judgments. *Personality and Social Psychology Bulletin, 13,* 478–489.

Fredrickson, B. L. (1998). What good are positive emotions? *Review of General Psychology, 2,* 300–319.

Fredricksson, B. L. (2001). The role of positive emotions in positive psychology: The broaden and build theory of positive emotions. *American Psychologist, 56,* 218–226.

Friedman, M., & Roseman, R. (1974). *Type A behavior and your health.* New York: Knopf.

Frijda, N. H. (1986). *The emotions.* Cambridge: Cambridge University Press.

Frijda, N. H. (2007). *The laws of emotion.* Mahwah, NJ: Erlbaum.

Frijda, N. H. (2007). *The laws of emotion.* Mahwah, NJ: Erlbaum.

Frijda, N. H. (1993). The place of appraisal in emotion. In N. H. Frijda (Ed.), *Appraisal and beyond. A special issue of Cognition and Emotion* (pp. 357–387). Hillsdale, NJ: Lawrence Erlbaum.

Frijda, N. H. (2007). *The laws of emotion.* Mahwah, NJ: Erlbaum.

Gallese, V. (2003). The roots of empathy: The shared manifold hypothesis and the neural basis of intersubjectivity. *Psychopathology, 36,* 171–180.

Gallese, V. (2011). Mirror neurons, embodied simulation, and the neural basis of social identification. *Psychoanalytic Dialogues, 19,* 519–536.

Gazzaniga, M. S., Ivry, R. B., Mangun, G. R., & Steven, M. S. (2009). *Cognitive neuroscience. The biology of the mind* (3rd ed.). New York: Norton.

George, J. M., & Brief, A. P. (1996). Motivational agendas in the workplace: The effects of feelings on focus of attention and work motivation. *Research in Organizational Behaviour, 18,* 75–109.

Goleman, D. (1995). *Emotional intelligence. Why it can matter more than IQ.* London: Bloomsbury.

Goleman, D. (1998). *Working with emotional intelligence.* New York: Bantam Books.

Gottman, J., & Declaire, J. (1997). *Raising an emotionally intelligent child: The heart of parenting.* New York: Simon & Schuster.

Grandey, A. A. (2000). Emotion regulation in the workplace: A new way to conceptualize emotional labor. *Journal of Occupational Health Psychology, 5,* 95–110.

Greenberg, L. S. (2011). *Emotion-focused therapy.* Washington, DC: American Psychological Association.

Greenberg, M. A., & Lepore, S. J. (2004). Theoretical mechanisms involved in disclosure. In I. Nyklicek, L. Temoshok, & A. Vingerhoets (Eds.), *Emotional expression and health* (pp. 43–60). New York: Brunner-Routledge.

Greenberg, M. A., Wortman, C. B., & Stone, A. A. (1996). Emotional expression and physical health: Revising traumatic memories or fostering self-regulation? *Journal of Personality and Social Psychology, 71,* 588–602.

Griffin, S., & Mascolo, M. F. (1998). On the nature, development, and function of emotions. In M. F. Mascolo & S. Griffin (Eds.), *What develops in emotional development*? (pp. 3–28). New York: Plenum Press.

Grolnick, W. S., Bridges, S. J., & Connell, J. P. (1996). Emotion regulation in two-year-olds: Strategies and emotional expression in four contexts. *Child Development, 67,* 928–941.

Gross, J. J. (1998). Antecendent- and response-focused emotion regulation: Divergent consequences for experience, expression, and physiology. *Journal of Personality and Social Psychology, 74,* 224–237.

Gross, J. J. (2002). Emotion regulation: Affective, cognitive, and social consequences. *Psychophysiology, 39,* 281–291.

Gross, J. J. (Ed.). (2007). *Handbook of emotion regulation.* New York: The Guilford Press.

Gross, J. J., & John, O. P. (2003). Individual differences in two emotion regulation processes: Implications for affect, relationships, and well-being. *Journal of Personality and Social Psychology, 85,* 348–362.

Gross, J. J., & Thompson, R. A. (2007). Emotional regulation: Conceptual foundations. In J. J. Gross (Ed.), *Handbook of emotion regulation* (pp. 3–26). New York: The Guilford Press.

Gross, J. J. (Ed.). (2007). *Handbook of emotion regulation.* New York: The Guilford Press.

Gross, J. J. (Ed.). (2007). *Handbook of emotion regulation.* New York: The Guilford Press.

Hammer, M. R., & Gudykunst, W. B. (1986). The influence of ethnicity and sex on social penetration in close friendships. *Journal of Black Studies, 17,* 418–437.

Harre, R., & Finlay-Jones, R. (1986). Emotion talk across times. In R. Harre (Ed.), *The social construction of emotions* (pp. 220–233). Oxford: Blackwell.

Harre, R. (1986). An outline of the social constructionist viewpoint. In R. Harre (Ed.), *The social construction of emotions* (pp. 2–14). London: Blackwell.

Harris, P. L. (1989). *Children and emotion.* Oxford: Blackwell.

Hart, S. (2009). *Den følsomme hjerne (The sensitive brain).* København: Hans Reitzels Forlag.

Hart, S. L., & Legerstee, M. (Eds.) (2010). *Handbook of jealousy.* Malden, MA: Blackwell Publishing Ltd.

Harter, S. (1983). Children's understanding of multiple emotions: A cognitive-developmental approach. In W. F. Overton (Ed.), *The relationship between social and cognitive development.* Hillsdale, NJ: Erlbaum.

Heelas, P. (1986). Emotion talk across cultures. In R. Harre (Ed.), *The social construction of emotions* (pp. 234–266). Oxford: Blackwell.

Hill, S. E., & Buss, D. M. (2008). The evolutionary Psychology of envy. In R. H. Smith (Ed.), *Envy, theory and research* (pp. 60–72). Oxford, UK: Oxford University Press.

Hjortsjø, C. (1969). *Man's face and mimic language.* Lund: Student Literature.

Hochschild, A. R. (1979). Emotion work, feeling rules, and social structure. *American Journal of Sociology, 85,* 551–575.

Hochschild, A. R. (1983). *The managed heart. The commercialization of human feeling*. Berkeley: The University of California Press.

Hochschild, A. R. (2003). *The managed heart. The commercialization of human feeling. Twentieth anniversary*. Berkeley: The University of California Press.

Hoffman, M. L. (1990). *Empathy and moral development*. Cambridge: Cambridge University Press.

Howard, D. J., & Gengler, C. (2001). Emotional contagion effects on product attitudes. *Journal of Consumer Research, 28,* 189–201.

Hsee, C. K., Hatfield, E., Carlson, J. G., & Chemtob, C. (1990). The effect of power on susceptibility to emotional contagion. *Cognition and Emotion, 4,* 327–340.

Hulsheger, U. R., Lang, J. W. B., Schewe, A. F., & Zijlstra, F. R. H. (2015). When regulating emotions at work pays off: A diary and an intervention study of emotion regulation and customer tips in service jobs. *Journal of Applied Psychology, 100,* 263–277.

Hulsheger, U. R., & Schewe, A. F. (2011). On the costs and benefits of emotional labor: A meta-analysis of three decades of research. *Journal of Occupational Health Psychology, 16,* 361–389.

Hupka, R. B. (1991). The motive for the arousal of romantic jealousy: Its cultural origin. In P. Salovey (Ed.), *The psychology of jealousy and envy* (pp. 252–270). New York: Guilford.

Van Ijzendoorn, M. H., & Sagi-Schwartz, A. (2008). Cross-cultural patterns of attachment: Universal and contextual dimensions. In J. Cassidy & P. R. Shaver (Eds.), *Handbook of attachment theory, research, and clinical applications* (2nd ed., pp. 880–905). New York: Guilford Press.

Illiescu, D., Illie, A., Ispas, D., & Ion, A. (2012). Emotional intelligence in personnel selection: Applicant reactions, criterion, and increment validity. *International Journal of Selection and Assessment, 20,* 347–358.

Isen, A. M., Daubman, K. A., & Nowicki, G. P. (1987). Positive affect facilitates creative problem solving. *Journal of Personality and Social Psychology, 52,* 1122–1131.

Isen, A. M., & Levin, P. F. (1972). The effect of feeling good on helping: cookies and kindness. *Journal of Personality and Social Psychology, 21,* 384–388.

Isen, A. M. (2004). Some perspectives on positive feelings and emotions: Positive affect facilitates thinking and problem solving. In A. S. R. Manstead, N. H. Frijda & A. Fischer (Eds.), *Feelings and emotions. The Amsterdam Symposium* (pp. 263–281). Cambridge: Cambridge University Press.

Izard, C. E. (1971). *The face of emotion*. New York: Appelton Century Crofts.

Izard, C. E. (1972). *Patterns of emotion: A new analysis of anxiety and depression*. New York: Academic Press.

Izard, C. E. (1991). *The psychology of emotions*. New York: Plenum Press.

Izard, C. E. (1993). Four systems for emotion activation: cognitive and non-cognitive processes. *Psychological Review, 1993,* 68–90.

Izard, C. E. (2007). Basic emotions, natural kinds, emotion schemas, and a new paradigm. *Perspectives in Psychological Science, 2,* 260–280.

Izard, C. E. (2009). Emotion theory and research: Highlights, unanswered questions, and emerging issues. *Annual Review of Psychology, 60,* 1–25.

Izard, C. E. (2009). Emotion theory and research: Highlights, unanswered questions, and emerging issues. *Annual Review of Psychology, 60,* 1–25.

Izard, C. E. (2009). Emotion theory and research: Highlights, unanswered questions, and emerging issues. *Annual Review of Psychology, 60,* 1–25.

Izard, C. E. (1972). Differential emotion theory and the empirical analysis of depression. In C. E. Izard (Ed.), *Patterns of emotion: A new analysis of anxiety and depression* (pp. 255–291). New York: Academic Press.

Izard, C. E., & Ackerman, B. P. (2000). Motivational, organizational, and regulatory functions of discrete emotions. In M. Lewis & J. M. Haviland-Jones (Eds.), *Handbook of emotions* (pp. 253–264). New York: The Guilford Press.

Izard, C. E. (1971). *The face of emotion*. New York: Appleton Century Crofts.

Izard, C. E. (2009). Emotion theory and research: Highlights, unanswered questions, and emerging issues. *Annual Review of Psychology, 60,* 1–25.

Izard, C. E. (1972). *Patterns of emotion: A new analysis of anxiety and depression*. New York: Academic Press. (b).

Izard, C. E., & Ackerman, B. P. (2000). Motivational, organizational, and regulatory functions of discrete emotions. In M. Lewis & J. M. Haviland-Jones (Eds.), *Handbook of emotions* (pp. 253–264)). New York: The Guilford Press.

Izard, C. E. (1991). *The psychology of emotions*. New York: Plenum Press.

John, O. P., & Gross, J. J. (2004). Healthy and unhealthy emotion regulation: Personality processes, individual differences, and life span development. *Journal of Personality, 72,* 1302–1333.

Johnson, E. H. (1990). *The deadly emotions*. New York: Praeger.

Joseph, D. L., Jin, J., Newman, D. A., & O'Boyle, E. H. (2015). Why does self-reported emotional intelligencer predict job performance? A meta-analytic investigation of mixed EI. *Journal of Applied Psychology, 100,* 298–342.

Kahneman, D. (2011). *Thinking, fast and slow*. New York: Farrar, Straus and Giroux.

Kahneman, D., & Krueger, A. B. (2006). Development in the measurement of subjective well-being. *Journal of Economic Perspectives, 20,* 3–24.

Kahneman, D., Krueger, A. B., Schkade, D. A., Schwartz, N., & Stone, A. A. (2004). A survey method for characterizing daily life experience: The day reconstruction method. *Science, 306,* 1776–1780.

Kemeny, M. E. (2003). The psychobiology of stress. *Current Directions in Psychological Science, 12,* 124–129.

Kemeny, M. E., & Shestyuk, A. (2008). Emotions, the neuroendocrine and immune systems, and health. In M. Lewis, J. M. Haviland-Jones, & L. Feldman Barrett (Eds.), *Handbook of emotions* (3rd ed., pp. 651–675). New York: Guilford.

Klineberg, O. (1954). *Social psychology*. New York: Holt.

Klinnert, M. D. (1984). The regulation of infant behavior by maternal facial expressions. *Infant Behavior & Development, 7,* 447–465.

Koole, S. L. (2009). The Psychology of emotion regulation: An integrative review. *Cognition and Emotion, 23,* 4–41.

Kopp, C., & Neufeld, S. J. (2003). Emotional development during infancy. In R. Davidson, K. Scherer, & H. H. Goldsmith (Eds.), *Handbook of affective science* (pp. 347–374). Oxford, UK: Oxford University Press.

Kring, A. M., & Werner, K. H. (2004). Emotion regulation and psychopathology. In P. Philippot & R. S. Feldman (Eds.), *The regulation of emotion (s* (pp. 359–386). Mahwah, New Jersey: Lawrence Erlbaum.

Krohne, H. W., Hock, M., & Kohlmann, C.-W. (1992). Coping dispositions, uncertainty and emotional arousal. In K. T. Strongman (Ed.), *International review of studies on emotion* (Vol. 2, pp. 73–96). New York: Wiley.

Lambie, J. A., & Marcel, A. J. (2002). Consciousness and the varieties of emotion experience: A theoretical framework. *Psychological Review, 109,* 219–259.

Larsen, R. J., & Buss, D. M. (2002). *Personality psychology*. New York: McGraw Hill.

Larsen, J. T., Berntson, G. G., Poehlmann, K. M., Ito, T. A., & Cacioppo, J. T. (2008) The psychophysiology of emotion. In M. Lewis, J. M. Haviland-Jones, & L. Feldman Barrett (Eds.), *Handbook of emotions* (3rd ed, pp. 180–195). New York: Guilford.

Lazarus, R. S. (1991). *Emotion and adaptation*. New York: Oxford University Press.

Lazarus, R. S., & Alfert, E. (1964). Short-circuiting of threat by experimentally altering cognitive appraisal. *Journal of Abnormal and Social Psychology, 69,* 195–205.

Lazarus, R. S. (1993). From psychological stress to the emotions: A history of changing outlooks. *Annual Review of Psychology, 44,* 1–21.

LeBon, G. (1960). *The crowd*. New York: Viking. (Original work published in 1895).

LeDoux, J. E. (1991). Emotion and the limbic system concept. *Concepts in neuroscience, 2,* 169–199.

LeDoux, J. E. (2000). Emotion circuits in the brain. *Annual Review of Neuroscience, 23,* 155–184.

LeDoux, J. E., & Phelps, E. A. (2008). Emotional networks in the brain. In M. Lewis, J. M. Haviland-Jones & L. Feldman Barrett (Eds.), *Handbook of emotions* (*3rd* ED., pp. 159–179). New York: Guilford.

Leach, C. W. (2008). Envy, inferiority, and injustice: Three bases of anger about inequality. In R. H. Smith (Ed.), *Envy, theory and research* (pp. 73–116). Oxford, UK: Oxford University Press.

Leff, J. (1973). Culture and the differentiation of emotional states. *British Journal of Psychiatry, 123,* 299–306.

Levine, L. J., & Pizarro, D. A. (2006). Emotional valence, discrete emotions, and memory. In B. Uttl, N. Ohta, & A. L. Siegenthaler (Eds.), *Memory and emotion* (pp. 37–58). Oxford: Blackwell Publishing.

Levy, R. I. (1973). *Tahitians: Mind and experience in the Society Islands*. Chicago: University Chicago Press.

Levy, R. I. (1984). Emotion, knowing, and culture. In R. A. Schweder & R. A. LeVine (Eds.), *Culture theory. Essays on mind, self, and emotions* (pp. 214–238). Cambridge: Cambridge University Press.

Lewis, M. (1993). The emergence of emotions. In M. Lewis & J. M. Haviland-Jones (Eds.), *Handbook of Emotions* (pp. 223–235). New York: The Guilford Press.

Lewis, C., & Mitchell, P. (Eds.). (1994). *Children's early understanding of mind*. Hillsdale, N.J: Lawrence Erlbaum.

Lewis, M. (2010). Loss, protest, and emotional development. In S. L. Hart & M. Legerstee (Eds.), *Handbook of jealousy* (pp. 27–39). Malden, MA: Blackwell Publishing Ltd.

Loewenstein, G. F., Hsee, C. K. W., & Welch, N. (2001). Risk as feelings. *Psychological Bulletin, 127,* 267–286.

Lutz, C. A. (1988). *Unnatural emotions. Everyday sentiments on a Micronesian atoll and Their challenge to Western theory*. Chicago: University of Chicago Press.

Lutz, C. A., & White, G. M. (1986). The anthropology of emotions. *Annual Review of Anthropology, 15,* 405–436.

Lyons, W. (1992). An introduction to the philosophy of the emotions. In K. T. Strongman (Ed.), *International review of studies on emotion* (Vol. 2, pp. 295–314). New York: Wiley.

MacLean, P. D. (1990). *The triune brain in evolution: Role of paleocerebral functions*. New York: Plenum.

Markus, H. R., & Kitayama, S. (1994). The cultural construction of self and emotion: Implications for social behavior. In S. Kitayama & H. R. Markus (Eds.), *Emotion and culture* (pp. 89–132). Washington, DC: American Psychological Association.

Martins, A., Ramalho, N., & Morin, E. (2010). A comprehensive meta-analysis of the relationship between emotional intelligence and health. *Personality and Individual Differences, 49,* 554–564.

Massumi, B. (2002). *Parables for the virtual: Movements, affect, sensation*. Durham, NC: Duke University Press.

Mastropieri, D., & Turkewitz, G. (1999). Prenatal experience and neonatal responsiveness to vocal expressions of emotion. *Developmental Psychobiology, 35,* 204–214.

Matsumoto, D., et al. (2008). Mapping expressive differences around the world. The relationship between emotional display rules and individualism versus collectivism. *Journal of Cross-Cultural Psychology, 39,* 55–74.

Matt, J. J. (2011). Current emotion research in history: Or, doing history from the inside out. *Emotion Review, 3,* 117–124.

Matthews, G., Zeidner, M., & Roberts, R. D. (2002). *Emotional intelligence. Science and myth*. Cambridge, Massachusetts: The MIT Press.

Maul, A. (2012). The validity of the Mayer-Salovey-Caruso emotional intelligence test. *Emotion Research, 4,* 394–402.

Mauss, I. B., & Gross, J. J. (2004). Emotion suppression and cardiovascular disease. In I. Nyklicek, L. Temoshok, & A. Vingerhoets (Eds.), *Emotional expression and health* (pp. 61–81). New York: Brunner-Routledge.

Mauss, I. B., & Robinson, M. D. (2009). Measures of emotion: A review. *Cognition and Emotion, 23,* 209–237.

Mayer, J. D., Salovey, P., & Caruso, D. R. (2002). *Mayer-Salovey-caruso emotional intelligence test user's manual*. Toronto, Canada: Multi-Health Systems.

Mayer, J. D., Salovey, P., & Caruso, D. R. (2004). Emotional intelligence: Theory, findings, and implications. *Psychological Inquiry, 15,* 197–215.

Mayer, J. D., Salovey, P., & Caruso, D. R. (2008). Emotional intelligence: New ability or eclectic traits? *American Psychologist, 63,* 503–517.

Mayo, F. (1933). *The human problems of an industrial civilization*. Cambridge, MA: Harvard.

McIntosh, D. (1996). Facial feed-back hypotheses: Evidence, implications, and directions. *Motivation and Emotion, 20,* 121–147.

McRae, R. R., & Costa, P. T. (1990). *Personality in adulthood*. New York: The Guilford Press.

Mead, M. (1935). *Sex and temperament in three primitive societies*. New York: William Morrow.

Meltzoff, A. N., & Moore, M. K. (1983). Newborn infants imitate adult facial gestures. *Child Development, 54,* 702–709.

Meltzoff, A. N., & Moore, M. K. (1983). Newborn infants imitate adult facial gestures. *Child Development, 54,* 702–709.

Meltzoff, A. N., & Moore, M. K. (1989). Imitations in newborn infants: Exploring the range of gestures imitated and the underlying mechanism. *Developmental Psychology, 25,* 954–962.

Mesquita, B., & Frijda, N. H. (1992). Cultural variations in emotions: A review. *Psychological Bulletin, 112,* 179–204.

Miller, S. M. (1987). Monitoring and blunting: Validation of a questionnaire to assess styles of information seeking under threat. *Journal of Personality and Social Psychology, 52,* 345–353.

Miranda, M., & Kihlstrom, J. F. (2005). Mood congruence in childhood and recent autobiographical memory. *Cognition and Emotion, 19,* 981–998.

Morris, J. A., & Feldman, D. C. (1996). The dimensions, antecedents, and consequences of emotional labor. *Academy of Management Review, 21,* 986–1010.

Morris, J. A., & Feldman, D. C. (1997). Managing emotions in the workplace. *Journal of Managerial Issues, 9,* 257–274.

Myers, L. B., & Derakshan, N. (2004). The repressive coping style and avoidance of negative affect. In I. Nyklicek, L. Temoshok, & A. Vingerhoets (Eds.), *Emotional expression and health* (pp. 169–184). New York: Brunner-Routledge.

Naring, G., Vlerick, P., & Van de Ven, B. (2012). Emotion work and emotional exhaustion in teachers: The job and individual perspective. *Educational Studies, 38,* 63–72.

Neal, D. T., & Chartrand, T. (2011). Embodied emotion perception: Amplifying and dampening facial feed-back modulates emotion perception accuracy. *Social Psychological and Personality Science, 2,* 673–678.

Niedenthal, P. M., Halberstadt, J., Margolin, J., & Innes-Ker, A. H. (2000). Emotional state and the detection of change in facial expressions of emotion. *Emotional Journal of Social Psychology, 30,* 211–222.

Niedenthal, P., Krauth-Gruber, S., & Ric, F. (2006). *Psychology of emotion*. New York: Psychology Press.

Nolen-Hoeksema, S., McBride, A., & Larson, J. (1997). Rumination and psychological distress among bereaved partners. *Journal of Personality and Social Psychology, 72,* 855–862.

Oatley, K., & Duncan, E. (1992). Incidents of emotion in daily life. In K. T. Strongman (Ed.), *International review of studies on emotion* (Vol. 2, pp. 249–294). New York: Wiley.

Oatley, K., & Jenkins, J. M. (1996). *Understanding emotion*. Oxford: Blackwell.

Oatley, K., & Johnson-Laird, P. N. (1987). Toward a Cognitive theory of emotions. *Cognition and Emotion, 1,* 29–50.

Oatley, K. (2004). *Emotions. A brief history*. Oxford: Blackwell.

Ochsner, K. N., Bunge, S. A., Gross, J. J., & Gabrielli, J. D. E. (2002). Rethinking feelings: An fMRI study of the cognitive regulation of emotion. *Journal of Cognitive Neuroscience, 14,* 1215–1229.

Øhman, A., & Soares, J. J. F. (1994). "Unconscious anxiety": Phobic responses to masked stimuli. *Journal of Abnormal Psychology, 103,* 231–240.

Olsson, A., & Phelps, E. A. (2004). Learned fear of "unseen" faces after Pavlovian, observational, and instructed fear. *Psychological Science, 15,* 822–828.

Olsson, A., & Phelps, E. A. (2007). Social learning of fear. *Nature Neuroscience, 10,* 1095–1102.

Ortony, A., Clore, G. L., & Collins, A. (1988). *The Cognitive structure of emotions*. New York: Cambridge University Press.

Panksepp, J. (2007). Neurologizing the psychology of affects: How appraisal-based constructivism and basic emotion theory can coexist. *Perspectives on Psychological Science, 2,* 281–296.

Panksepp, J., & Biven, L. (2012). *The archaeology of mind*. New York: Norton.

Panksepp, J. (1991). Affective neuroscience: a conceptual framework for the neurobiological study of emeotions. In K. Strongman (Ed.), *International review of studies in emotions* (Vol. I, pp. 55–99). Chichester: Wiley.

Panksepp, J. (2004a). Affective consciousness: Core emotional feelings in animals and humans. *Consciousness and Cognition, 14,* 30–80.

Panksepp, J. (2004b). Basic affects and instinctual emotional systems of the brain. In A. S. R. Manstead, N. Frijda, & A. Fischer (Eds.), *Feelings and emotions. The Amsterdam Symposium* (pp. 174–193). Cambridge, UK: Cambridge University Press.

Panksepp, J., & Biven, L. (2012). *The archaeology of mind*. New York: Norton.

Pardilla, P. P., & Calvete, Z. E. (2015). A test of the vulnerability-stress model with brooding and reflection to explain depressive symptoms in adolescence. *Journal of Youth and Adolescence, 44,* 860–869.

Parkinson, B., & Totterdell, P. (1999). Classifying affect-regulation strategies. *Cognition and Emotion, 13,* 277–303.

Parkinson, B., & Totterdell, P. (1999). Classifying affect-regulation strategies. *Cognition and Emotion, 13,* 277–303.

Parrott, W. G., & Smith, R. H. (1993). Distinguishing the experiences of envy and jealousy. *Journal of Personality and Social Psychology, 64,* 906–920.

Peace, K. A., & Porter, S. (2004). A longitudinal investigation of the reliability of memories for trauma and other emotional experiences. *Applied Cognitive Psychology, 18,* 1143–1159.

Pekrun, R., & Frese, M. (1992). Emotions in work and achievement. In C. I. Cooper & I. T. Robertson (Eds.), *International review of industrial and organizational psychology* (Vol. 7, pp. 153–200). Chichester: John Wiley.

Pennebaker, J. W. (1990). *Opening up: The healing power of confiding in others*. New York: William, Morrow.

Pennebaker, J. W., & Beall, S. (1986). Confronting a traumatic event: Toward an understanding of inhibition of behavior. *Journal of Personality and Social Psychology, 49,* 1427–1433.

Pennebaker, J. W. (1989). Confession, inhibition, and disease. In L. Berkowitz (Ed.), *Advances in experimental social psychology* (Vol. 22, pp. 211–244). Orlando, FL: Academic Press.

Peristiany, J. G. (1974). *Honour and shame*. Chicago: Chicago University Press.

Pessoa, L., & Adolphs, R. (2010). Emotion processing and the amygdala: From a "low road" to "many roads" of evaluating biological significance. *Nature Reviews Neuroscience, 11,* 773–782.

Pessoa, L. (2013). *The cognitive-emotional brain. From interactions to integration*. Cambridge, MA: The MIT Press.

Petrides, K. V., & Furnham, A. (2000). On the dimensional structure of emotional intelligence. *Personality and Individual Differences, 29,* 313–320.

Petrides, K.V., & Furnham, A. (2001). Trait emotional intelligence: Theory, findings, and implications. *Psychological Inquiry,* 197–215.

Phelps, E. A. (2005). The interaction of emotion and cognition: Insights from studies of the human amygdala. In L. Feldman Barrett, P. M. Niedenthal, & P. Winkielman (Eds.), *Emotion and consciousness* (pp. 51–66). New York: The Guilford Press.

Piola-Merlo, A., Hartel, C., Mann, L., & Hirst, G. (2002). How leaders influence the impact of affective events on team climate and performance in R&D teams. *The Leadership Quarterly, 13,* 561–581.

Plutchik, R. (1980). *Emotion, A psychoevolutionary synthesis*. New York: Harper & Row.

Pons, F., Harris, P. L., & De Rosnay, M. (2004). Emotion comprehension between 3 and 11 years: Developmental periods and hierarchical organization. *European Journal of Developmental Psychology, 1,* 127–152.

Porges, S. W. (2011). *The Polyvagal theory. Neurophysiological foundations of emotions, attachment, communication and self-regulation*. New York: W. W. Norton.

Porter, R. E., & Samovar, L. A. (1998). Cultural influences on emotional expression: Implications for intercultural communication. In P. A. Andersen & L. K. Guerrero (Eds.), *Handbook of communication and emotion* (pp. 451–472). San Diego, CA: Academic Press.

Pugh, S. D. (2001). Service with a smile: Emotional contagion in the service encounter. *The Academy of Management Journal, 44,* 1018–1027.

Reiche, E. M. V., Morimoto, H. K., & Nunes, S. O. V. (2006). Stress and depression-induced immune dysfunction: Implications for the development and progression of cancer. *International Review of Psychiatry, 17,* 515–527.

Rime, B., Herbette, G., & Corsini, S. (2004). The social sharing of emotion: Illusory and real benefits of talking about emotional experiences. In I. Nyklicek, L. Temoshok, & A. Vingerhoets (Eds.), *Emotional expression and health* (pp. 29–42). New York: Brunner-Routledge.

Rime, B., Mesquita, B., Philippot, P., & Boca, S. (1991). Beyond the emotional event: Six studies on the social sharing of emotion. *Cognition and Emotion, 5,* 435–465.

Rime, B., Paez, D., Kanyangara, P., & Yzerbyt, V. (2011). The social sharing of emotions in interpersonal and in collective situations: Common psychosocial consequences. In I. Nyklicek, A. J. J. M. Vingerhoets, & M. Zeelenberg (Eds.), *Emotion regulation: Conceptual and clinical issues* (pp. 147–164). New York: Springer.

Rivers, S. E., Brackett, M. A., Katulac, N. A., & Salovey, P. (2007). Regulating anger and sadness: An exploration of discrete emotions in emotion regulation. *Journal of Happiness Studies, 8,* 393–427.

Rizzolatti, G., Fadiga, L., Gallese, V., & Fandassi, L. (1996). Premotor cortex and the recognition of motor actions. *Cognitive Brain Research, 3,* 131–141.

Rohleder, N., Chen, E., Wolf, J. M., & Miller, G. E. (2008). The psychobiology of trait shame in young women: Extending the social self-preservation theory. *Health Psychology, 27,* 523–532.

Rosen, H. J., & Levenson, R. W. (2009). The emotional brain: Combining insights from patients and basic science. *Neurocae, 15,* 173–181.

Rothbart, M. K., Ziaie, H., & O'Boyle, S. G. (1992). Self-regulation and emotion in infancy. In N. Eisenberger & R. A. Fabes (Eds.), *Emotion and its regulation in early development. New Directions in Child Development* (No. 55, pp. 7–23). San Francisco: Jossey Bass.

Rozin, P., Lowry, L., Imada, S., & Haidt, J. (1999). The CAD triad hypothesis: A mapping between three moral emotions (contempt, anger, disgust) and three moral codes (community, autonomy, divinity). *Journal of Personality and Social Psychology, 76,* 574–586.

Rozin, P., Haidt, J., & McCauley, C. R. (2008). Disgust. In M. Lewis, J. M. Haviland-Jones, & L. Feldman Barrett (Eds.), *Handbook of emotions* (3rd ed., pp. 757–776). New York: Guilford.

Russell, J. A. (1991). Culture and the categorization of emotions. *Psychological Bulletin, 110,* 426–450.

Russell, J. A. (1994). Is there universal recognition of emotion from facial expression? A review of cross-cultural studies. *Psychological Bulletin, 115,* 102–141.

Russell, J. A. (2003). Core affect and the psychological construction of emotion. *Psychological Review, 110,* 145–172.

Saarni, C., Campos, J. J., Camras, L. A., & Witherington, D. (2006). Emotional development: Action, communication, and understanding. In N. Eisenberg, W. Damon, & R. Lerner (Eds.), *Handbook of Child Psychology* (6th ed., Vol. 3, pp. 226–300). New York: Wiley.

Salovey, P., & Mayer, J. D. (1989). Emotional intelligence. *Imagination, Cognition, and Personality, 9,* 185–211.

Sapolsky, R. M. (1994). *Why zebras don't get ulcers*. New York: Freeman and Company.

Schachter, S., & Singer, J. (1962). Cognitive, social and physiological determinants of emotional state. *Psychological Review, 69,* 379–399.

Scherer, K. R. (1988). *Facets of emotion: Recent research*. Hillsdale, NJ: Lawrence Erlbaum.

Scherer, K. R. (2001). Appraisal considered as a process of multilevel sequential checking. In K. R. Scherer, A. Schorr, & T. Johnstone (Eds.), *Appraisal processes in emotion* (pp. 92–120). Oxford: Oxford University Press.

Scherer, K. R., Wallbott, H. G., & Summerfield, A. B. (Eds.). (1986). *Experiencing emotion: A cross-cultural study*. Cambridge, UK: Cambridge University Press.

Scherer, K. R. (1993). Studying the emotion-antecedent appraisal process: An expert systems approach. In N. H. Frijda (Ed.), *Appraisal and beyond. A special issue of Cognition and Emotion* (pp. 325–356). Hillsdale, NJ: Lawrence Erlbaum.

Schoeck, H. (1969). *Envy*. Indianapolis: Liberty Fund.

Schore, A. N. (1994). *Affect regulation and the origin of the self: The neurobiology of emotional development*. Hillsdale, NJ: Erlbaum.

Schutte, N. S., Malouff, J. M., Hall, L. E., Haggerty, D. J., Cooper, J. T., Golden, C. J., et al. (1998). Development and validation of a measure of emotional intelligence. *Personality and Individual Differences, 25,* 167–177.

Schwartz, N. (2001). Feelings as information: Moods influence judgments and processing strategies. In T. Gilovich, D. Griffin, & D. Kahnemann (Eds.), *The psychology of intuitive judgment* (pp. 534–547). Cambridge: Cambridge University Press.

Selye, H. (1956). *The stress of life*. New York: McGraw Hill.

Shaffer, D. R. (2009). *Social and Personality Development* (6th ed.). Boston, Ma.: Cengage Learning.

Siegling, A. B., Saklofske, D. H., & Petrides, K. V. (2015). Measures of ability and trait emotional intelligence. In G. J. Boyle, D. H. Saklofske, & G. Matthews (Eds.), *Personality and social psychological constructs* (pp. 381–414). Amsterdam: Elsevier.

Simon, H. A. (1967). Motivational and emotional controls of cognition. *Psychological Review, 74,* 29–39.

Smith, C. A., & Ellsworth, P. C. (1985). Patterns of cognitive appraisal in emotion. *Journal of Personality and Social Psychology, 48,* 813–838.

Smith, R. H., & Kim, S. H. (2007). Comprehending envy. *Psychological Bulletin, 133,* 46–64.

Smith, R. H. (1991). Envy and the sense of injustice. In I. P. Salovey (Ed.), *The psychology of jealousy and envy* (pp. 79–99). New York: Guilford.

Spielberger, C. D. (1972). Conceptual and methodological issues in research on anxiety. In D. Spielberger (Ed.), *Anxiety: Current trends in theory and research* (Vol. 2, pp. 481–493). New York: Academic Press.

Sroufe, L. A. (1996). *Emotional development*. Cambridge: University of Cambridge.

Sroufe, L. A. (1996). *Emotional development*. Cambridge: University of Cambridge.

Sroufe, L. A. (1996). *Emotional development*. Cambridge: University of Cambridge.

Stearns, C., & Stearns, P. (1986). *Anger: The struggle for emotional control in America's history*. Chicago, Ill.: University of Chicago Press.

Stern, D. (1977). *The first relationship*. London: Open Books.

Stipek, D. (1995). The development of pride and shame in toddlers. In J. P. Tangney & K. W. Fischer (Eds.), *Self-conscious emotions* (pp. 237–254). New York: The Guilford Press.

Strack, F., Martin, L., & Stepper, S. (1988). Inhibiting and facilitating conditions of the human smile: A nonobtrusive test of the facial feedback hypothesis. *Journal of Personality and Social Psychology, 54,* 768–777.

Strongman, K. T. (1996). *The Psychology of emotion. Theories of emotion in perspective* (4th ed.). New York: Wiley.

Susskind, J. M., Lee, D. H., Cusi, A., Feiman, R., Grabski, W., & Anderson, A. K. (2008). Expressing fear enhances sensory acquisition. *Nature Neuroscience, 11,* 843–850.

Tangney, J. P. (1995). Shame and guilt in interpersonal relationships. In J. P. Tangney & K. W. Fischer (Eds.), *Self-conscious emotions* (pp. 114–139). New York: The Guilford Press.

Tarde, G. (2003). *The laws of imitation*. New York: Henry Holt Inc. (Original work published in 1890).

Taylor, G. J. (1997a). Affects and alexithymia in medical illness and disease. In G. J. Taylor, R. M. Bagby, & J. D. A. Parker (Eds.), *Disorders of affect regulation* (pp. 216–247). Cambridge: Cambridge University Press.

Taylor, G. J. (1997b). Introduction. In G. J. Taylor, R. M. Bagby & J. D. A. Parker (Eds.), *Disorders of affect regulation* (pp. 1–6). Cambridge: Cambridge University Press.

Thompson, R. A. (1994). Emotion regulation: A theme in search of a definition. In N. A. Fox (Ed.), *The development of emotion regulation. Monographs for the Society for Research in Child Development, 59*(2–3), 25–52.

Thrift, N. (2008). *Non-representational theory: Space, politics, and affect*. London: Routledge.

Tomkins, S. S. (1962). *Affect, imagery, consciousness. The positive affects* (Vol. 1). New York: Springer.

Tomkins, S. S. (1963). *Affect, imagery, consciousness. The negative affects* (Vol. 2). New York: Springer.

Tracy, J. L., & Robins, R. W. (2007). The nature of pride. In J. L. Tracy, R. W. Robins, & J. P. Tangney (Eds.), *The self-conscious emotions* (pp. 263–282). New York: The Guilford Press.

Turner, J. H. (2009). The sociology of emotions: Basic theoretical arguments. *Emotion Review, 1,* 340–354.

Turner, J. H., & Stets, J. E. (2005). *The sociology of emotions*. Cambridge: Cambridge University Press.

Turnipseed, D. L., & Vandewaa, E. A. (2012). Relationship between emotional intelligence and organizational citizenship behavior. *Psychological Reports, 110,* 899–914.

Vikan, A., Dias, M., & Nordvik, H. (2009). Perceived efficiency and use of strategies for emotion regulation. *Psychological Reports, 104,* 455–467.

Vikan, A., Johnsen, H., Moen, T., Hassel, A. M., & Rugseth, A. (2010a). A norwegian normation of cook's internalized shame scale (ISS). *Nordic Journal of Psychiatry, 64,* 196–202.

Vikan, A., Kårstad, S. B., & Dias, M. (2013). Young Brazilian and Norwegian children's concepts of strategies and goals for emotion regulation. *Journal of Early Child Research, 11,* 63–77.

Vikan, A., Rugseth, A., & Hassel, A. M. (2010b). Outpatients' ratings of the use and efficiency of emotion regulation strategies. *Nordic Psychology, 62,* 50–66.

Vikan, A., Rugseth, A., & Hassel, A. M. (2010). Outpatients' ratings of the use and efficiency of emotion regulation strategies. *Nordic Psychology, 62,* 50–66.

Vikan, A. (2006). Empati (Empathy). In M. Tetzchner, E. Grindheim, J. Johannessen, D. Smørvik, & V. Ytterland (Eds.), *Biologiske forutsetninger for kulturalisering (Biological prerequisites for culturalization* (pp. 331–350). Psykologisk Institutt: Universitetet i Oslo.

Vikan, A., Dias, M., & Nordvik, H. (2009). Perceived efficiency and use of strategies for emotion regulation. *Psychological Reports, 104,* 455–467.

Vikan, A., Dias, M., & Nordvik, H. (2009). Perceived efficiency and use of strategies for emotion regulation. *Psychological Reports, 104,* 455–467.

Visser, V. A., van Knippenberg, D., van Kleef, G. A., & Wisse, B. (2013). How leader displays of happiness and sadness influence follower performance: Emotional contagion and creative versus analytical performance. *The Leadership Quarterly, 24,* 172–188.

Walker-Andrews, A. S., & Dickson, L. R. (1997). Infants' understanding of affect. In S. Hala (Ed.), *The development of social cognition* (pp. 161–186). Hove, East Sussex: Psychology Press.

Wallbott, H. G., & Scherer, K. R. (1988). How universal and specific is emotional experience? Evidence from 27 countries. In K. R. Scherer (Ed.), *Facets of emotions* (pp. 31–56). Hillsdale NJ: Erlbaum.

Wallbott, H. G., & Scherer, K. R. (1986). How universal and specific is emotional experience? Evidence from 27 countries on five continents. *Social Science Information, 25*, 763–795.

Watson, J. B., & Raynor, R. (1920). Conditioned emotional reactions. *Journal of Experimental Psychology, 3,* 1–14.

Webb, T. L., Miles, E., & Sheeran, P. (2012). Dealing with feeling: A meta-analysis of the effectiveness of strategies derived from the process model of emotion regulation. *Psychological Bulletin, 138,* 775–808.

Weiskrantz, L. (1956). Behavioral changes associated with ablation of the amygdaloid complex in monkeys. *Journal of Comparative and Physiological Psychology, 49,* 381–391.

Werner, K. H., & Gross, J. J. (2010). Emotion regulation and psychopathology: A conceptual framework. In I. A. M. Kring & D. M. Sloan (Eds.), *Emotion regulation and psychopathology* (pp. 13–37). New York: The Guilford Press.

Wetherell, M. (2012). *Affect and emotion*. London: Sage.

Wikan, U. (1990). *Managing turbulent hearts; A Balinese formula for living*. Chicago: University of Chicago Press.

Williams, K. E., Chambless, D. L., & Ahrens, A. (1997). Are emotions frightening? An extension of the fear of fear construct. *Behaviour Research and Therapy, 35,* 239–248.

Winkielman, P., Berridge, K. C., & Wilbarger, J. L. (2005). Unconscious affective reactions to masked happy versus angry faces influence consumption behavior and judgment of value. *Personality Social Psychology Bulletin, 31,* 121–135.

Wittstein, I. S., et al. (2005). Neurohumoral features of myocardial stunning due to sudden emotional stress. *New England Journal of Medicine, 352,* 539–548.

Yank, G. R., Bentley, K. J., & Hargrove, D. S. (1993). The vulnerability-stress model of Schizophrenia: Advances in psychosocial treatment. *American Journal of Orthopsychiatry, 63,* 55–69.

Yerkes, R. M., & Dodson, J. D. (1908). The relation of strength to rapidity of habit formation. *Journal of Comparative and Neurological Psychology, 18,* 459–482.

Yiend, J. (2010). The effects of attention on emotion: a review of attentional processing of emotional information. *Cognition and Emotion, 24,* 3–47.

Yuille, J. C., & Cutshall, J. L. (1986). A case study of eyewitness memory of a crime. *Journal of Applied Psychology, 71,* 291–301.

Zajonc, R. B. (1980). Feeling and thinking: Preferences need no inferences. *American Psychologist, 35,* 151–175.

Zapf, D. (2002). Emotion work and psychological well-being. A review of the literature and some conceptual considerations. *Human Resource Management Review, 12,* 237–268.

Author Index

A. Vikan, *A Fast Road to the Study of Emotions*,
DOI 10.1007/978-3-319-52313-2

Subject Index

A. Vikan, *A Fast Road to the Study of Emotions*,
DOI 10.1007/978-3-319-52313-2

MIX
Papier aus verantwortungsvollen Quellen
Paper from responsible sources
FSC® C105338

If you have any concerns about our products,
you can contact us on
ProductSafety@springernature.com

In case Publisher is established outside the EU,
the EU authorized representative is:
Springer Nature Customer Service Center GmbH
Europaplatz 3, 69115 Heidelberg, Germany

Printed by Libri Plureos GmbH
in Hamburg, Germany